CONCILIUM

concilium 1997/5

THE RETURN OF THE PLAGUE

Edited by

José Oscar Beozzo and Virgil Elizondo

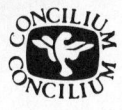

SCM Press · London
Orbis Books · Maryknoll

Published by SCM Press Ltd, 9–17 St Albans Place, London N1
and by Orbis Books, Maryknoll, NY 10545

Copyright © Stichting Concilium

English translations © 1997 SCM Press Ltd and Orbis Books, Maryknoll

All rights reserved. No part of this publication may be reproduced, stored in a retrieval system, or transmitted, in any form or by any means, electronic, mechanical, photocopying or otherwise, without the prior written permission of Stichting Concilium, Prins Bernhardstraat 2 6521 A B Nijmegen. The Netherlands

ISBN: 0 334 03046 3 (UK)
ISBN: 1 57075 130 7 (USA)

Typeset at The Spartan Press Ltd, Lymington, Hants
Printed by Biddles Ltd, Guildford and King's Lynn

Concilium Published February, April, June, October, December

Contents

Editorial: The Return of the Plague   vii
    José Oscar Beozzo and Virgil Elizondo

I · Plagues Today

God and the Evil of this World. Forgotten, Unforgettable Theodicy   3
    Johann Baptist Metz

Plagues: Definition and Overall View   9
    Gaspar Mora

The Social Construction of Plagues   18
    John H. Simpson

Evil in the Free Market Mentality   24
    Jung Mo Sung

II · Biblical/Theological Interpretation

'Neither he nor his parents have sinned . . .' Guilt and Exclusion   35
    Hermann Häring

Plagues in the Bible   45
    Pablo Richard

Job: 'Even when I cry out "Violence!" I am not answered'   55
    Elsa Tamez

Leprosy: Untouchables of the Gospel and of Today   63
    Justin S. Upkong

The Apocalyptic Beast: The Culture of Violence   71
    Walter Wink

III · The Challenge of the Plague Experience

Plague and its Human Price: Albert Camus, *The Plague*   81
    Norbert Mette

The Christian Ethic: Help or Hindrance? MARCIANO VIDAL	89
Seeds of Hope ZILDA ARNS NEUMANN	99
Contributors	109

Editorial

The Return of the Plague

Decades of giddy technological and scientific progress, advances in the fields of medicine and public health, with the eradication of endemic diseases and the control of epidemics, are being cancelled out by the uncontrollable rise of new diseases such as HIV and Ebola, together with the unexpected return of other virtually extinct ones such as cholera, yellow fever, malaria and measles.

It is as though the Horsemen of the Apocalypse had suddenly burst back, like lightning from a clear sky, with their fourfold following of catastrophe: war, famine, disease, death. Reactions of fear, panic, or the rebirth of old mechanisms of self-protection, seeking the guilty or scapegoats, creating new social stigmas, exclusions and ghettoes, are once more feeding popular imagination with visions of the Plagues of Egypt or the Apocalypse and thoughts of God's punishment for the sins of the human race. Our placid confidence in the advances and efficacy of science and medicine, our blind faith in technological and scientific progress, have been destroyed. The world is once again peopled with demons and monsters from the tormented and disturbing canvases of Hieronymus Bosch or the science-fiction creations of TV and cinema.

The epidemics of the past and the plagues of today connote the unexpected and uncontrollable aspects of human life, reviving tendencies to assign blame for these incomprehensible misfortunes. Reversals of fortune, suffering and poverty were formerly attributed to sin and linked to divine punishment, as challenges to the quality of our religious understanding and the capacity of theology to provide answers to the anguished cry of the Jobs of today. At the present time, entire populations of undesirables and untouchables for ethnic, social or religious reasons, and multitudes of so-called 'economic refugees', are being excluded or even exterminated under a wide variety of different pretexts or excuses. What is the meaning of all this? What is the challenge such situations pose to us as human beings and Christians?

This issue of *Concilium* seeks to face these disturbing questions by, first, mapping out the plagues besetting our world today: social plagues translating into hunger, poverty and exclusion, and raining down on the populations of the Third World, of Africa in particular, but also translating into the unemployment, suicides, drugs, depression and xenophobia afflicting the developed capitalist societies. We are equally concerned not to ignore the plagues of organized crime, ethnic and religious conflicts, environmental pollution, insecurity and impoverishment affecting the countries of Eastern Europe and other regions of the world. Gaspar Mora provides this initial overall view of the phenomenon.

This appreciation forces us to listen to the cry of the innocent victims of these processes and to take up their anguished challenge to the silence and impotence of God, to the indifference or sluggishness of Christians and churches in facing up to these new challenges, to the failure of states to assure them a minimum of security and hope. It also obliges us not to shrink from the question underlying the whole situation: 'If God is good, how to explain so much evil in the world?' John Baptist Metz reviews the drama of Job and points up the course followed by Jesus, who looked straight at the sufferings and not at the sins of others. But there is also the strange logic informing the market economy, which calls good what was formerly considered evil, and evil what were hard-sought values of societies called civilized. Many of its theorists view unemployment, cuts in social benefits and in public spending on health, education and old-age pensions as necessary sacrifices to establish a new pattern of growth. The assurance of full employment, the implementation of social policies designed to eradicate poverty, do away with economic exclusions and reduce social inequalities are seen as an affront to the freedom of the market and blocks to competition and modernization, which alone are capable of ensuring economic growth and the ultimate happiness and well-being of those who are part of it. 'Outside the market there is no salvation' is presented by Jung Mo Sung as the supreme law prohibiting, in the name of its principles, any struggle against our modern economic and social plagues.

Plagues as a phenomenon beyond our control by the same token provoke a complex social response, with the need to dissect not only their psychological structure and mechanisms, but also their economic, social and political ones, and the support they find in religious explanations and theological constructs. The second block of articles investigates this disturbing world of punishment, blame and exclusion, with the article by H. Häring, which pleads for a firm option for the victims, based on Jesus' observation, faced with the man born blind, that 'Neither he nor his parents have sinned'. The Apocalypse, Exodus and the book of Job furnish the kernel of biblical reflection on plagues in the articles by Pablo Richard, Elsa Tamez and Walter Wink, while Justin Ukpong explores the relationship between the lepers and untouchables of Jesus' time and the various 'leprosies' of today.

The final block of articles examines the challenge posed by the experience of plagues. Marciano Vidal analyses the help that Christian ethical reflection can bring to the difficult questions faced by persons and societies afflicted by plagues. He also faces up to the obstacles placed by a certain type of moral stance in the way of solving problems or diminishing human suffering and anguish. The inspiring contribution by Zilda Arns Neumann shows the seeds of hope sown by an exemplary pastoral child-care initiative in Brazil and how, with few resources, many of the plagues afflicting the most vulnerable sectors of humanity, women and children, can be tackled. Norbert Mette analyses a classic of contemporary literature, Albert Camus' *The Plague*, read as a metaphor for extreme situations, a city devastated by plague. Camus paints the dramatic scenario of human impotence in the face of evil and the struggle of some to overcome it, even against all hope.

Translated by Paul Burns

José Oscar Beozzo
Virgil Elizondo

I · Plagues Today

God and the Evil of this World. Forgotten, Unforgettable Theodicy

Johann Baptist Metz

The topic of this issue, 'The Return of the Plague', finally confronts theology with the question which in scholastic terminology is discussed under the heading of 'theodicy'. How does talk of God – note, not some postmodern invented 'God', but the remembered God of the biblical traditions, of the God of Abraham, Isaac and Jacob who is also the God of Jesus – relate to the experiences of evil, suffering and wickedness in the world, in 'his' world? Attempts at such a theological answer, a theological explanation of evil in the world, have been and are manifold. They cannot be pursued in detail within the framework of this text, nor should they be[1] – especially as my starting point is that there is no 'answer', no 'solution', to this question by means of which theology could settle it once and for all, provided that the question is put properly. This conclusion governs my approach. But anyone who speaks of God in the sense of the biblical traditions encounters the question of theodicy. It is and remains *the* eschatological question. What does it mean?

Exodus theodicy – Job theodicy

This issue of *Concilium* picks up a word which is familiar to us from the biblical traditions, the so-called 'plagues of Egypt'. In the book of Exodus these plagues are described in detail and a 'justification' is also given for this visitation of misery on Egypt. This is a divine punitive action against the Pharaoh of Egypt with his sinfully hardened heart, who is preventing the liberating exodus of Israel. Evil as a punishment for sin: down to the present day this is a recurrent motif in 'answers' to the question of theodicy. However, already in the biblical traditions themselves there is a counter-story to this Exodus theodicy, namely the Job theodicy. This Job theodicy makes it quite clear (and in the relevant narrative passages even finds the approval of God himself for this) that the plagues which fall on Job, his suffering and his misfortune, have nothing to do with his sin or with his failure before God. Here a just and innocent man is suffering! So there is no causal connection between suffering and sin.

The eschatological question

In order to take account of the complexity of the theodicy question, I do not propose to start directly from the 'plagues', from the evils of this world, but from what I would like to call here the 'human history of suffering'.[2] In my view this category of the history of suffering undermines the familiar distinction between physical evils (natural catastrophes, epidemics, illnesses . . .) and 'moral evil' (guilt, evil); however, above all it prevents an over-hasty ontologization of the problem, of the kind known to us from the history of theology and philosophy, especially in all dualistic or quasi-dualistic attempts at an explanation, e.g. in the theodicy of Gnosticism and the Gnostic relapse in Christianity.[3] Now if we begin with the 'human history of suffering', we shall no longer misunderstand theodicy as the attempt at a belated and to some degree defiant 'justification of God' by theology in the face of the evil, suffering and wickedness in the world. Moreover we shall recognize that theodicy is concerned, indeed is exclusively concerned, with the question how it is possible to talk of God at all in the face of the abysmal history of suffering in a world which we acknowledge in faith to be God's creation. This question may not be either eliminated or over-answered by theology; it is, as I have already said, *the* eschatological question. Theology does not work out any all-reconciling answer to it but continually seeks a new language and praxis in order to make it unforgettable.

Two fundamental reservations

Of course there are objections to such a 'weak' conception of theodicy. Here I shall discuss – briefly – two fundamental reservations, namely 1. objections which are made in the name of reason and 2. objections which are made in the name of Christian doctrine.

1. Does not this conception contradict a principle of human reason which is expressed, for example, in Ockham's razor: *entia sine ratione non sunt multiplicanda* (entities are not to be multiplied without reason)? Applied to our topic, is it not necessary on rational grounds finally to drop and forget a question to which, it is granted, there can be no answer? But what if one day human beings could defend themselves against the

unhappiness in the world only with the weapon of forgetfulness, if they could build their happiness only on the uncompassionate forgetfulness of the victims, on a culture of amnesia? What if only time heals all wounds (and one day even the wounds which bear the name of Auschwitz)? If that happens, on what does resistance to the senselessness of suffering in the world feed? What inspires an attentiveness to the suffering of others and the vision of a new and greater justice? What remains if this cultural amnesia is complete? The human being? What human being? An appeal to the self-preservation of the human in this instance seems to me to be highly abstract. It derives not least from an anthropology which has long bidden farewell to the question of evil and the 'perspective of theodicy' in human history and which forgets that not only the individual human being but also the 'idea' of humanity is vulnerable, indeed can be destroyed.

2. Does not the 'weak' conception of theodicy presented here contradict the theological understanding of Christianity as this has developed over centuries? Is not Christianity the successful response to and also the stilling of that question of theodicy which accompanied the history of the faith of Israel in the form of lament, cry and insatiable expectation – in the Psalms, in Job, in Lamentations, in many passages in the prophetic books? Is not christology, is not above all Christian soteriology, the answer to the question of the history of human suffering in God's good creation?[4]

But even the christology of Christians does not lack eschatological unrest. Not only Israel has constantly moved in an eschatological 'landscape of cries';[5] as is well known, the New Testament, the biography of early Christianity, ends with a cry, with a cry which now has a christological point, though in the meantime this has usually been silenced in a mythical or idealist-hermeneutical way. In his article 'Why Does God Let Us Suffer?',[6] Karl Rahner mentions an account by Walter Dirks, which has often been quoted since, of a meeting with Romano Guardini, who already had the marks of death on him. This is an account in which it becomes dramatically clear how much the question of theodicy constantly disturbs the whole of Christian doctrine: 'The one who experiences it will not forget what the old man on his sick bed entrusted to him. He would not only allow himself to be asked questions at the Last Judgment but would also himself ask questions: he confidently hopes that the angel would not refuse to give him a true answer to the question which no book, not even scripture, no dogma and no magisterium, no "theodicy" and theology, not even his own, has been able to answer for him, "Why, God, this fearful way round to salvation, the suffering of the innocent, guilt?"' Why the burden and excessive demands of the human history of suffering? Why guilt? This question remains. Why sin? This 'first' question of theodicy does not derive from a typically intellectual cult of questioning, which would indeed be most remote from the sufferers themselves. No vague speculative questions, but passionate personal questions are part of that experience of God about which Christians have had to learn time and again. And this above all because the mysticism which Jesus lived and taught is not really a mysticism of closed eyes but a mysticism of open eyes, which obligates us to a heightened perception of the suffering of others.

Jesus' first gaze

Christianity began as a community which remembered and told stories in the footsteps of Jesus, whose first gaze was not directed to the sin of others but to the suffering of others. This sensitivity to the suffering of others, this heeding of the suffering of others – including the suffering of enemies – in Jesus' own action lies at the centre of that 'new way of living' which is associated with him. It is the most convincing expression of that love which Jesus entrusted to us and asked of us when – completely in line with his Jewish heritage – he invoked the unity of love of God and love of neighbour.

There are parables of Jesus with which he told himself into human memory. One of the best-known parables is that of the 'Good Samaritan', with which he illustrates this love. Here (in the imagery of an archaic provincial society) it is the one who fell among thieves who is disregarded by the priest and the levite 'in the interest of higher things'. Those who look for 'God' as Jesus understands God do not know 'any higher interest' to excuse them here. This authority of the sufferer is the only authority in which the authority of the God who judges manifests itself in the world for all human beings (Matt. 25.31–46). Conscience constitutes itself in obedience to it, and what we call its voice is our reaction to a visitation by this suffering of others.

However, at a very early stage Christianity lost its elemental sensitivity to suffering. The question of justice for innocent sufferers which disturbs the biblical traditions was restated too quickly and transformed into the question of redemption for the guilty. Thus theology believed that it could draw the sting of the question of theodicy. The question of suffering found itself in a soteriological circle. Christianity transformed itself from a religion which was primarily sensitive to suffering into a religion which was primarily sensitive to sin. The focus of attention was no longer on the suffering of the creature but on its guilt. That paralysed the elemental sensitivity to the suffering of others and darkened the biblical vision of the great justice of God, though according to Jesus this had to apply to all hunger and thirst.

Questions about the adventure of theodicy

Our concern here has been above all with a background reflection on the question of God and the evils of this world, on fate and the enduring significance of the question of theodicy in Christianity. But is not this concentration on the question of theodicy too much characterized by resignation and evasion? Are there any open ears in Christianity to the heightened sensitivity for the suffering of others? Should not religion protect us from the pain of negativity? If it does anything at all, does it not serve the triumph of the 'positive', the optimizing of the chances of survival? And finally, is not the sensitivity to suffering addressed here an attitude which is very difficult for young people in particular to achieve and show to others? Youth and theodicy: is not that *a priori* a combination doomed to failure?

I can attempt to answer this only with a counter-question. To whom should one entrust the attention addressed here which is paid to the suffering of others, an attitude of empathy which is boundless ('There is no suffering in the world which does not concern us'[7])? Of whom should one require the adventurous notion of being there for others before one receives anything from them? To whom could one offer the 'other way of living' thus indicated? To whom, I ask myself, if not to young people in particular? Have we completely forgotten that Christianity once began as a revolt of the youth within the Jewish world of the time?

Has Christianity possibly already grown too old for the sensitivity to suffering which is required by Jesus? Is the refusal of a theodicy really the sign of a living Christianity? Is it not rather the sign of a Christianity which is growing old? The older Christianity becomes, the more 'affirmative' it seems to become, the more closed it seems to be, passing over the refractory features of creation. A sense of the misfortune of others is withering away; the steadfastness of faith is insidiously becoming the steadfastness of bewilderment. Anyone who now still has questions, passionate questions, for God is suspected of either loosing the tongue of doubt or propagating a cult of negativity. For me the specifically Christian form of fundamentalism is reflected in such an attitude. Such a kind of fundamentalism is a symptom of ageing, which does not really dare to look the negative features of the world in the face. It has lost the first gaze of Jesus.

Translated by John Bowden

Notes

1. In his brief work 'Why Does God Let Us Suffer?', *Theological Investigations* 10/2, London and New York 1973, 450–66x, Karl Rahner offers a brief but convincing criticism of the common attempts to make sense of the suffering and evil of this world.

2. For this encounter see my text 'Die Rede von Gott angesichts der Leidengeschichte der Welt', *Stimme der Zeit* 1992/5. This text has since appeared in English (*Critical Inquiry*, 1994).

3. See here for example the investigations by H. Blumenberg in *Säkularisierung und Selbsbehauptung*, Frankfurt 1974. Theodor W. Adorno has pointed out that concepts of theodicy which make use of an ontological argument end up in an ontology of the torment of creation. Cf. now J. A. Zamora's work on Adorno, *Krise – Kritik – Erinnerung*, Münster 1995.

4. For the aporias of the classical position of Augustine and contemporary attempts to respond to the question of theodicy with talk of the 'suffering God' cf. all the contributions in J. B. Metz (ed.), *'Landschaft aus Schreien.' Zur Dramatik der Theodizeefrage*, Mainz 1995. See also W. Gross and K.-J. Kuschel, *'Ich schaffe Finsternis and Heil'. Ist Gott verantwortlich für des Übel?*, Mainz 1992.

5. A formulation of Nelly Sachs.

6. See n. 1 above.

7. A formulation of Peter Rottländer.

Plagues: Definition and Overall View

Gaspar Mora

We start with a distressing observation: that in our world there is a proliferation of seriously inhuman situations invading our life and society with the uncontrollable force of destructive currents. Some of these varied phenomena can be listed as: AIDS, unemployment, the growth of the 'fourth world', droughts and famines, sex tourism, criminal religious fundamentalism, violence in the great conurbations, psychological depression, refugees, traffic accidents, child abuse, female genital mutilation . . . The list could be extended but is already giddying. These are the new plagues afflicting humankind.

Politics and ethics *ad usum* are helpless in the face of phenomena of such magnitude. These require new reflection and new approaches appropriate to the new challenges they pose. As a first contribution, this article attempts to define the facts we are dealing with, to describe their characteristics and the elements of which they are composed. As a start, we need to ask whether it is possible to formulate these elements.

1. The framework for a definition

The very fact of posing the problem is in itself symptomatic, corresponding to two characteristics of the present moment. The first of these is the globalization of human experience: it is now clear that limited and partial views are of no use; anthropological questions are raised on a world-wide scale and have to be understood from this characteristic. On our subject, partial experiences of evil combine with all others to form a whole in time and space. It is no longer possible to take an individual or partial view of these phenomena: the globalizing character of our mentality sees them as plagues.

The second characteristic is more important – our postmodern sensibility. We live in a particular time, when the great anthropological and ethical options of modernity – scientific progress, valuation of freedom, pluralism and tolerance – are still valid, but the climate has changed: it is marked by two negative accents, disenchantment with the great discourses of enlightened modernism and a hidden but lively terror in the face of a future with no clear direction. This climate has made the definition of our evils, our 'plagues', possible. Disillusion with regard to the great projects of freedom, democracy, scientific progress and universal justice creates the sensibility needed to detect the misfortunes crowding in on us, which have taken over, at least partly, from the just, free and human world promised by the great projects of modernity.

This framework should put us on our guard against an excessively 'catastrophist' posing of the problem. Our postmodernity shows us the deceit of modernity; disillusion and disenchantment show, at least partly, the elements of 'illusion' and 'magic' in the great modern discourses – that is, deceit on human beings and their possibilities. Observing our plagues brings us back to the true reality of the human situation. In fact, many of our plagues are no more than an accentuation, or a simple present-day observation, of age-old afflictions, which may well have been more serious. If we look on AIDS as a plague, it is probably no worse than the bubonic plague or tuberculosis of past centuries, and the same could be said of so many present-day versions of plagues that have always afflicted humankind: wars with all their cruelties, abortion, child sexual abuse, genocides, and so on. Our current disenchantment can lend present-day plagues a special note of horror that can be stupefying. Darkness coming after a light shining into our eyes seems darker than it is. We need to re-draw our picture of 'real people' if we are to make an accurate assessment of our plagues, without denying them, but also without considering them a sort of ultimate apocalyptic scourge.

2. Characteristics of the new plagues

The word 'plague' evokes the biblical chastisements of Exodus and the Apocalypse, and recalls historical experiences of epidemics, diseases against which humanity seemed powerless, or swarms of harmful creatures. Today's events do not quite share these characteristics. They do, however, share common elements that justify calling them 'plagues': they are scourges that affect the whole planet, are destructive, operate on a wide scale, and are above all progressive, all-embracing, invasive, uncontrollable and unstoppable. One way or another, the misfortunes that concern us are experienced as evils that increase, invade us, are beyond our control, and this was true of the traditional plagues. The present-day ones, nevertheless, have their own special characteristics, which give them a new gravity of their own.

(a) Human intervention: the effects of freely-made decisions

This is probably the most distinctive feature enabling the term 'plague' to be applied to the present-day versions and setting them apart from the traditional ones. With the latter, human beings were victims of a vast collective scourge against which they could do nothing: epidemics, famines, diseases . . . Today, on the other hand, we apply the word destructive and invasive currents in which we and our freely-made decisions are implicated: the waves of refugees, abortion, the sexual abuse of children, unemployment, ecological disasters, traffic accidents, and many other examples that could be given, are terrible and destructive evils but not ones that crush humanity from outside; they proceed rather from their own choices.

Even the present plagues that most resemble the traditional ones – the AIDS and Ebola viruses, but also the residues of malaria and tuberculosis – fall under this new aspect. The clearest example is AIDS, one of the worst of modern scourges. The disease is not spread by some magic or unknown means but by such identifiable means as sexual relations and blood contact. These fall right into the field of conscious human decision-making, and it is precisely this that gives AIDS its special horror. But something similar could be said of other epidemic diseases to the extent that they are spread through lack of proper hygiene or prophylaxis, both of which humanity can supply.

This is what gives our modern plagues a special, disturbing, dramatic note. The very fact that we can make fairly accurate statistical forecasts of the number of unemployed next year, the number of deaths from drug overdoses or road accidents, the number of practitioners and victims of sex tourism, gives modern plagues a note of heart-rending suffering. They seem to be mechanisms advancing relentlessly, spreading destruction and pain, but the most unbearable pain comes precisely from the fact that these mechanisms are made unstoppable by a series of human decisions, taken in the vast dark sphere of our freedom.

In this, too, present-day plagues evoke something very typical of our postmodern sensibility: terror of ourselves. It is instructive to follow the process of such an important and so obscure an anthropological phenomenon as fear. We have always experienced terror, have attributed it to a thousand causes, and have sought refuge from it in a thousand solutions. The ethos of modernity denounced the occult and dark occurrence of fear in many human experiences, including some of the most sublime, and declared our ancestral terrors banished by the advance of science, psychological studies, and human cultural maturity. Here, too, postmodernity has seen the great modern projects of human fulfilment tumble. We are not looking simply at the demise of great hopes but at the re-emergence of terror — no longer, though, terror of dark or divine forces, but of ourselves, on account of the terrible destructive force of our bad intentions or mere disregard. The growth in sexual abuse of children, or of pollution, or of the inhuman growth of mega-conurbations in the Third World, or the degradation of marginalized and excluded groups, produces an overpowering terror at the possibilities for destruction stemming from our own decisions, perhaps above all when these are taken in a climate of despairing unawareness. This fact probably has to become a hermeneutic criterion for understanding the ultimate meaning of our terrors and the deceit of attributing them to external and occult forces; at bottom we are afraid of our own limitations and of our own human wickedness. In the light of the plagues raining down on us, we have to admit that this fear is not a pathological deception; it is real.

(b) An evil that destroys humanity

The evil aspect of today's plagues can be summed up under this double anthropological heading: human beings are both their cause and their victims. Let us reflect on this second aspect, which can be subdivided into two secondary headings. First, we need to stress the world-wide cultural consensus that human life and well-being constitute the criterion for an ethical evaluation of any event, including our plagues. These plagues are an evil phenomenon in that they destroy human beings and human lives, degrade our dignity as individuals or as groups, dehumanize individuals, groups and peoples. The cultural consensus needs to be emphasized as forming one of the most positive elements in our present-day world, the fruit of the clearly anthropocentric orientation of modernity. In effect, attempts to work out a universal course of action, on both the political and ethical levels, are based on the good of each person and of all human groups. We also need to stress the consensus between Christian thought and this basic modernist orientation. Vatican II consecrated the essentially anthropological emphasis of Christian experience, thereby marking a new direction in the difficult relationship between Christian faith and modern thought, through doing away with the disjunction between the gift of God and human freedom that had poisoned the whole course of modernity. This peaceable accord in seeing present-day plagues as an evil is another sign of the global consensus on taking humankind as the ethical criterion.

But just as they are a symptom of the common modern experience, so also the plagues are a symptom of its complex ambiguity. Putting forward human well-being as our criterion involves posing the anthropological question in our plural world, even within the church. Though they rest on a common base, diverse, even highly divergent concepts of human life and fulfilment are evident today, always within a pluralist outlook that denies any pretension to global truth to a specific current of thought.[1] Applying anthropological pluralism to our concern here in the light of our previous considerations, we see that phenomena such as abortion, the 'fourth world', unemployment or divorce call for very distinct judgments. Here too, the new plagues are a field for experimentation in our new outlook. Christian thinking, for its part, is also fully involved in the coordinates of the conflict.

Within one same anthropological confession different accents are placed on the value given to human freedom, law and order, sexuality, the autonomy of conscience, the distribution of resources. To take just one example: the proliferation of methods of birth regulation can be viewed, depending on one's anthropological perspective, as either a true plague of degradation of human sexuality, or as a positive indication of human dominion over the laws of our nature. And the same could be said of other controversial phenomena such as abortion, unemployment, or the inequality among societies.

The ecological question merits special attention in this section. It is clear that ecological disasters should be viewed as real plagues. And it can be said that we assess such disasters as evil also for anthropological reasons. With few exceptions, natural processes are not seen as sacred in themselves but in their close relationship with human life and progress. At the root of ecological sensibility is an intimate conviction of the indissoluble unity between the good of nature and the good of humankind itself, which forms part of nature and stands in a delicate relationship to it. But conflict begins the moment we start to define – in theory and practice – the requirements imposed by respect for natural processes. There are different ecological concepts, varying with different concepts of human well-being, achievement and progress. Anthropological pluralism also affects differing views of ecological misfortunes: they can be seen as unacceptable plagues or as necessary, even good, conditions for human growth.

(c) Plagues as a new subject for adverse moral judgment

There is no doubt that modernity introduced the social element into our understanding of human life. The human phenomenon cannot be grasped in all its complexity without attending to the intimate relationship between individuals and society, so that culture and cultures now form an essential part of the definition of what it means to be human. The ethical repercussions of this fact are enormous. Traditional morality held to a very individualistic understanding of behaviour. Now, reflection on moral decisions has to examine in depth the delicate tension between the individual and the social dimension inherent in them.

In considering the morally evil subject of this article, the study by

Antonio Moser on the social aspect of sin is highly relevant.[2] He distinguishes three steps in the slow process towards true understanding of the social dimension to human sinfulness: the social dimension in personal sins, collective sin and structural sin. He analyses these phenomena and stresses what is particular to each, insisting on the need to avoid equating them with one another. Understanding each stems from the same social outlook but accentuates distinct aspects marking the process of a growing clear-sightedness on the still little-studied fact of the social dimension to wrong human decisions. Now the concept of 'plague' needs to be introduced as a new category in the analysis of what is socially morally wrong.

According to Moser, accenting the 'social dimension of sins' lays stress on the 'repercussion of personal sins on others, and even on human history', in a process going from the personal to the interpersonal, community and social dimensions. 'Collective sin' refers more to 'a people and an episodic situation of disregard or culpable collaboration. The field involved is the political-ideological one and the accent is placed only on persons, though considered collectively.' 'Structural sin', on the other hand, refers to 'a complex of mechanisms at once social, political, economic, ideological and even religious that, even supposing the human element to be ultimately responsible, function with a certain autonomy once established. The accent is not placed on persons or groups, though these are not excluded. The accent is on the mechanisms.'

'Plague' constitutes a new aspect of social wrong. It does not refer to the cause – as the concept of structural sin does – but rather to the effect; not so much as a simple evil for which there is a social responsibility – as in the concept of collective sin – but stressing its proper characteristics as examined above: its world-wide scale, its invasive and unstoppable growth, and, above all, its character as destructive of human life and dignity through the free choices made by human beings, the means of bringing about these very invasive and destructive effects.

It is also enlightening to emphasize another difference: the first concepts studied – the social dimension of personal sin, collective sin, structural sin – respond to an objective and cold analysis of the social dimensions of human wrongdoing. This analysis, however, is objective and cold only in appearances. Fundamentally, it derives from a sensibility very proper to modernity, which analyses evil in the firm conviction that it can be confronted and overcome. Moderns are not neutral but optimists; they are convinced they can conquer the evil they uncover. By contrast, the idea of 'plague' derives from a clearly postmodern analysis. Postmoderns are not neutral but pessimists. They project their disappointment and pain on to the concept of 'plague'; plagues – AIDS, child pornography, arms deals with the Third World, unemployment, divorce – are an invasive, destructive evil, advancing precisely through freely-taken human decisions, in an advance that is despairingly unstoppable. The concept of 'plague' enshrines the most desolating experiences of postmodernity, the failure of the great discourses and terror of an undefined future.

3. Types of plagues

The concept of 'plague' I have tried to define includes very disparate experiences of evil. It is time to attempt a classification, but difficult to find a single criterion in the midst of such diversity, so I propose a broad classification as at least offering some clarification of the concept itself.

(a) Plagues originating in nature

This is the aspect that accords most closely with the traditional conception of 'plague'. The most typical example is AIDS: this is a natural serious evil – an illness – wide-scale, destructive, invasive, unstoppable. This example is a good sample for understanding the complexity of this first category, 'natural plagues'. I have already stressed that it is not transmitted by means unknown or that we cannot tackle, but basically through sexual relations and blood contact, means that are theoretically under human control. The fact of human intervention is essential to the new understanding of plague. This is why this view can include, besides AIDS, other naturally-occuring evils which are invasive, uncontrollable, and to some extent subject to human intervention: the Ebola virus, malaria, tuberculosis, drought, famine.

All these plagues have their origin in natural processes but all suppose some type of human intervention. In the case of AIDS this is direct and necessary for the transmission of the disease; in the case of other diseases – malaria, tuberculosis, cholera, yellow fever, some of which seemed vitually extinct but are returning in plague proportions – the human intervention can be seen as indirect, since their spread depends largely on lack of hygiene, nourishment, or prophylaxis, things currently within the ambit of human possibilities. Droughts and famines affecting certain regions with catastrophic results also fall into this category: they demonstrate a terrible human disregard, since it is now technically possible to confront and palliate these natural misfortunes, to the point where extraordinarily ambitious programmes are mounted to resolve far less serious problems. Some natural scourges, however, fall outside this category as completely beyond human intervention: earthquakes, floods, or swarms of harmful insects or animals.

(b) Age-old human plagues

Our present mentality has opened our eyes to many phenomena loaded with inhumanity that have always scourged human existence. It is not our age that has invented sexual abuse of young girls or mass deportations. They have been known from all time, but the confused conviction that a final happy outcome would be found through science or democracy has probably veiled the terrible nature of such inhumanities. The contribution of our age has been that after so much discourse and effort, including the spilling of so much blood, inhumanities are still with us, recurring as plagues with no sight of a resolution.

Let us list some of these ever-renewed disgraces on humanity: wars, exiles, cruelty to the vanquished, religious fundamentalisms, the systematic slaughter of enemy groups, prostitution, child labour, inhuman treatment of women, the caste system, racisms of all types – exclusive, absorbing, destroying. We note with horror so many present evils that have their origin in an ancestral, implacable inhumanity – which our age does no better than repeat, even adding new degrees of inhumanity.

I believe we also need to include some other practices stemming from ages past but until recently unperceived by most people. Their discovery as practices that have been going on for centuries and are still being repeated gives them a special note of horror: female genital mutilation, child prostitution, specially cruel legal punishments meted out even to children, hidden enmities and vendettas among various social groups . . . Our age has taken note of their existence, scale and persistence. Knowledge of them can seem to be a secondary question set beside the gravity of the facts themselves, but this is not so. This is not a simple knowledge, but one loaded with significance, public, commentated, dominant. In our age information is more than pure information; in the case that concerns us here it is a becoming conscious of terrible evils, caused by human inhumanity, implacably repeated, unstoppable. It is another form of experiencing the horror we feel at our human nature and the challenge it poses to us.

(c) New plagues

Many of our present plagues are new phenomena, mostly linked to the life-style of our society, with all the elements that go to make it up: accidents on the road and at work, pockets of urban deprivation, the influx into massive conurbations in the Third World, air and water pollution, unwanted children, unemployment, psychological depression and suicides, waves of emigration to wealthy countries, corruption on a grand scale, drugs, sex tourism, child prostitution, traffic in babies, terrorism, violence, daily insecurity, mafias of all kinds . . .

These are plagues that very much belong to our present world. They raise the question of the level of inhumanity that characterizes our society, a question formulated often and which goes beyond the scope of this article. At the very least, they denote a known and most lamentably human practice, and one that has on that account been with us always: the utilization of whatever situation by the sinful human mind to create news situations of inhumanity, degradation, destruction, in the name of interests that cannot be confessed.

Conclusion

At the beginning of this article I stressed that our postmodern sensibility has opened our eyes to the seriousness of the plagues afflicting our world, and I noted that this very fact should put us on our guard against an excessively 'catastrophist' and apocalyptic view of the evils that we have seen to exist. Perhaps part of this article has seemed to lean towards catastrophe; this is due to the seriousness of the subject, which poses major challenges to ethics, politics, theology, the church. At the very least we should be grateful for the sensibility that has made us so conscious of the real state of affairs, however serious it might be, without therefore falling into the trap of thinking that 'any period in the past was better'. Knowledge of reality is always good. Now we have to understand it as fully as we can and respond to the challenge it poses.

Translated by Paul Burns

Notes

1. I have studied these categories in my article 'La situació actual de la moral. Vers la segons recerca del fonament', *Rev. Cat. de Theol.* XVII, 1992, 157–92. Spanish summary in *Selec. de Teol*, 34, 1995, 143–55.

2. A. Moser, 'Pecado estructural', in F. Compagnoni, G. Piana, S. Privitera, M. Vidal (eds.) *Nuevo Diccionario de Teología Moral*, Madrid 1992.

The Social Construction of Plagues
John H. Simpson

A plague is both a constructed phenomenon – a human experience that is interpreted in a symbolic universe of meaning – and a biophysical reality – an event in a human population that raises the risk of impairment or destruction of persons and their bodies beyond ordinary, expected levels. While plague as an interpreted construction and plague as a biophysical event are analytically distinct, it is impossible to separate them in the flow of human life. They form a system.

A plague's meaning is always relative to the cultural resources where it occurs: a population's mythologies, theories of the empirical world, techniques and orientations to strangers and others. The biophysical event of plague occurs where one population of organisms (including humans) preys on another population (including humans). Thus war, plunder and pillage (macro-parasitism) and virulent disease (micro-parasitism) are forms of plague.

Sometimes macro- and micro-parasitic forms of plague are entwined. American troops fighting in Quebec during the Revolutionary War (1776–1783) outnumbered the British two to one. Nevertheless, the Americans were forced to retreat when smallpox invaded and decimated their ranks. It spared the British, who had been inoculated against the disease. Some say that smallpox delivered Canadians from United States citizenship!

Near the end of the twentieth century the memory of virulent disease-based plague has grown dim in popular and historical consciousness, especially in the affluent West, where medical science, organized public health and wealth provide an infrastructure that minimizes the presence of infectious disease. However, new forms of disease such as HIV still raise the spectre of plague, induce collective fear, and lead to the social construction of the diseased, stigmatized other. Furthermore, new forms of 'plague' have appeared such as the child-abuse panic in North America that seems to be linked to changes in family structure, changes in the participation rates and roles of women in the work force, and the construction of TV and in the newspapers of widespread social problems imputed to human intimacy.[1]

New forms of disease such as HIV affect both rich and poor populations alike on a global basis. In recent years old diseases such as malaria and cholera have reappeared with the force of plague among some populations in the Third World and developing countries. Poverty, unemployment, poor housing conditions in big cities and the general unwillingness of states to invest in public health and prevention programmes put millions of humans at risk as the old diseases reassert themselves among the world's poor at the end of the twentieth century.

Old and new plagues require an understanding of the 'epidemiology of representations'.[2] What images of plague circulate in human culture? Do they have a fundamental structure or logic? Where should the line be drawn, today, in the construction of the plague-ridden other? At what point do benefits such as the avoidance of disease or social 'infection' outweigh the human costs of such constructions – rejection, stigma, isolation, social death and, sometimes, real death? Answers to these questions begin with an examination of disease-based plagues whose effects – despite the forgetfulness of modernity – are deeply etched in human culture.

Some images of disease-based plague

The social construction of disease-based plague depends in the first place on the occurrence of a publically visible infection in a population. Where there are many cases of an easily transmitted disease that almost always kills those whom it infects, a classic plague exists. Rapid death underscores the perception of plague. It is probable that the Black Death in fourteenth-century Europe was a form of bubonic plague that led to death only one day after exposure and infection.

A plague, obviously, cannot occur (and, thus, be constructed) unless a population is exposed to infection. However, where outbreaks are frequent and a significant number survive, it is not likely that the disease will be perceived as a plague. Should infection provide immunity for survivors, a disease will be constructed as an ordinary childhood malady. If they are exposed, the children of immune adults may be infected, but their parents will not develop the disease. The infected children who survive form the next generation of immune, reproductive adults.

Where an often fatal, contagious disease infects a population and there are survivors (the disease is endemic) and the population encounters another population without previous experience of the disease, a plague will occur. The classic example is the spread of smallpox by the Spanish to the New World in the sixteenth century. The disease attacked the previously unexposed indigenous populations with epidemic force, causing high rates of death while hardly touching the conquering Spaniards.

In the common European manner of the day that Spaniards interpreted the pestilence as a sign of divine displeasure. Lacking any experience with epidemic disease and recognizing the extraordinary powers of all deities, the Amerindian populations tended to accept that interpretation. That the Spaniards were not struck down by smallpox but the native populations were may have had a role in the conversion of the native populations. Placating the God of the Spaniards (who, after all, had saved most of *them*) was a way of avoiding divine wrath and, thereby, preventing disease.[3]

Where effective control in the form of prevention or cure (or both) exists, the perception of virulence will be diminished, but sometimes at great human cost. Prevention may involve the construction and isolation of the diseased other as in quarantine. The labelling and segregation of the diseased other inevitably creates a deviant subject.

Plague and misplaced analogy

Measures taken to prevent the spread of disease may, themselves, be forms of destructive parasitism. Modern science provides an understanding of disease and its control that through erroneous analogy has on occasion increased the spread of disease rather than preventing it. Bubonic plague broke out in India in 1896. Measures that had been taken earlier in the century when cholera was epidemic and that were effective – segregation, hospitalization, disinfection and the inspection of travellers and goods in transit – were imposed by the British colonial administration. The sewers of Bombay were flushed regularly and houses suspected of harbouring the disease were disinfected, often in a destructive manner. Despite these measures the disease persisted.

By 1898 bubonic plague was known to be endemic in certain rat populations and there was speculation that it was transmitted to humans through flea bites, but the British proceeded as if the scientifically-based actions that prevented cholera would also curb bubonic plague. At best the measures had no effect, while stigmatizing a portion of the population – the lower classes believed to harbour the disease – and destroying their shelter. At worse they spread the disease. When sewers were flushed, rats infested with disease-bearing fleas fled to the streets.[4]

The dominant British classes along with other Western elites in the nineteenth century believed fervently in the efficacy of scientifically-based public health measures. Bubonic plague, however, is not cholera, and the effective, scientifically constructed means for dealing with the latter were, simply, magic when used on the former, an unfortunate application of a misguided analogy.

The construction of plague in tradition

Ironically, scientifically-based practices may fail and, indeed, may make things worse until the true science of a disease is established. On the other hand, practices associated with traditional stories or myths can be effective against disease. Thus Marcellus, saint and bishop of Paris in the fifth century, was credited by the hagiography of Merovingian Gaul with miraculously taming a dragon before the assembled people of Paris and banishing it from the region. There was a metonymous complex of dragons, snakes, water, floods, epidemic disease, drainage and bishops in the early Middle Ages that makes sense of the story as a narrative of 'public health' in the circumstance of epidemic malaria.[5]

Torrential rains in medieval Gaul caused floods that sometimes bore a horde of snakes driven from their dens by the surging waters. Epidemic malaria frequently followed a flood and was attributed to the figure of a dragon, a transposed snake whose noxious, fetid breath and other putrid emissions were thought to be a source of disease. (Stinking swamps, among other places, were often deemed to be the home of dragons.) By banishing the dragon, Marcellus would have been perceived as restoring health in Paris – not an unlikely outcome if he were responsible for drainage schemes. Early mediaeval bishops were, in fact, known to have taken up secular responsibilities for various public works including fortifications, dams and the continuation of Roman systems of drainage that prevented malaria.

Modernity and macro-parasitism

Dragons were a plague in early mediaeval Gaul. Those who slew or banished them got rid of disease. Scientific discourse enables us today to see the rhetorical equivalence of banishing dragons and draining swamps and appreciate the real, salubrious effects underlying some traditional stories. Tragically, scientific discourse had also been used to construct disastrous equivalence in modern times, a macro-parasitic plague where humans became vermin and science-based extermination led to a method for killing them.

Some Nazi propaganda with a documentary gloss dwelt on the connection between dirt, lice, rats, insects and disease and the need for cleanliness and modern sanitation at home and in industry. Germany was presented as a nation that was taking vigorous measures to cleanse itself thoroughly of dirt, vermin and disease with the help of modern scientific practices, including gas fumigation.[6]

There was a mad, propaganda-induced leap in Hitler's Germany from real vermin and insects to the insinuation of human equivalents – Jews, gypsies, 'defectives', homosexuals – in the taken-for-granted understandings of everyday life. Millions met the same fate in the Nazi gas chambers as the insects and rats that were so effectively eliminated by modern fumigation methods. Perhaps, that was *the* plague of the twentieth century.

The general social logic of plague

The social construction of plague – at least in the broad tradition of Western thought from early Christian times to the present – invokes the assimilation of events and agents to the dual categories of good/evil and purity/danger. The form of the logic underlying the construction of plagues is the same whether the frame of reference is theological or scientific. The event of plague arises from a malevolent or dangerous source (for example, human frustration of the will of God; an invasion of microbes) and can only be overcome by salutary practice (for example, God's delivering acts; quarantine and disinfection).

Problems arise in the modern circumstance from the misapplication of science, as in the Indian plague of 1896 or from the conflation of moral, social and scientific categories that makes the other vermin or an outcast as in the Holocaust or the contemporary construction by some of AIDS as an affliction that is *caused* by homosexuality. Science nevertheless can and does reveal the 'truth' of disease-based plague and enables us to take effective measures against it within variable limits depending on the disease. Yet these measures should always be tempered by contextualizing them within an analysis of the social logic of the interpretation of plague lest purity/danger be confused with good/evil and the other be constructed as an undesirable, dispensable element in a population, that is, as no more than a part of 'negative' 'standing-reserve',[7] and, as a consequence, be destroyed socially or materially.

Notes

1. J. H. Simpson, 'Organized Disclosures in Contemporary America: The Dedifferentiation of the Public Sphere and the Secularization of Modernity', in A. Shupe and B. Misztal (eds.), *Prophetic Religions in the 21st Century*. Westport, Connecticut and London 1997.
2. D. Sperber, 'Anthropology and Psychology: Towards an Epidemiology of Representations', *Man*, ns 20, 1985.
3. W. H. McNeil, *Plagues and Peoples*. Garden City, New York 1976.
4. R. Chandavarkar, 'Plague Panic and Epidemic Politics in India, 1896–1914', in T. Ranger and P. Slack (eds.), *Epidemics and Ideas: Essays on the Historical Perception of Pestilence*, Cambridge 1992.
5. P. Horden, 'Disease, Dragons and Saints: The Management of Epidemics in the Dark Ages', in ibid.
6. P. Cohen, director, *Architecture of Doom (Untergängens Arkitektur)*, produced and distributed by the Swedish Film Institute and others, Stockholm, Sweden 1989.
7. M. Heidegger, *The Question Concerning Technology and Other Essays*, New York 1977.

Evil in the Free Market Mentality

Jung Mo Sung

1. The strange logic of the market

'Wall St Celebrates Rise in Jobless.'[1] This headline from a major Brazilian newspaper is a typical example of the new mentality that dominates the market. Unemployment has ceased to be an economic and social evil and become, in many cases, an economic benefit. So, over the last few years, major corporations have made great efforts to introduce 'downsizing' programmes to reduce the numbers of their workforce, and the more they make redundant, the higher their share value rises, enriching their shareholders and executives. The pride and strength of companies no longer resides in the number of their employees but in the number of workers they can remove from their employment. This number serves as an index of increased efficiency and productivity, today's absolute economic criterion.

Those not accustomed to this strange logic of the market will find it difficult to understand this 'celebration'. This difficulty stems not only from their scant knowledge of economics, but from the fact that there has been a profound shift in the way of judging unemployment and other social problems. In the past, unemployment was always seen as an economic and social scourge. It was a scourge often impossible to foresee and difficult to control, the fruit of economic cycles, bad management, wars, or natural disasters – a sort of 'social plague', and, as such, an evil to be combatted. For a long period, economic policy after the Second World War made maintaining a low level of unemployment one of its prime objectives. Inspired by Keynesian theories, states intervened in the economy to generate employment and advocated social policies designed to mitigate the consequences of unemployment and reduce social inequality.

Today, on the other hand, high levels of unemployment are viewed as inevitable, the fruit of the new technological revolution and of economic globalization. Even the social exclusion of a significant section of humanity, the most glaring social fact of our day, no longer moves society. This social insensitivity shows that unemployment and social exclusion are no longer regarded as social problems but as individual ones, and as a social cost, a sacrifice worth making for the fantastic technological progress supplied by the free-market system. Therefore, the main objective of present-day economic policies is control of inflation, no longer job-creation and reduction in social inequality.

2. The market and the theology of sin

In order to understand this huge transformation a little better, we need to go back to the 1970s. At the beginning of that decade, Europe and the United States found themselves faced with a major economic crisis, characterized by a rise in inflation and unemployment coupled with economic recession – 'stagflation'. This crisis deeply shook the optimism born of the longest period of growth and economic expansion the world had ever known, following the Second World War. This growth was interpreted by neo-classical economists as the natural fruit of the market, conceived as a harmonious and balanced system that 'naturally' generated economic growth. This optimistic concept, born of a mechanistic view of the world, led the neo-classicists to stop worrying about the problems of economic fluctuations and unemployment, as classical economists had done. Keynesian economists themselves shared this mechanistic view of the world and the economy with neo-classical ones. The difference between them consisted in the fact that the Keynesians believed that state spending played an important role in the process of generating higher employment.

When a crisis such as that of the 1970s occurs, of such magnitude that it is impossible to deny its existence, and puts the basic consensus of society in check, we have to find new explanations for its causes if we are to be able to find means of overcoming it. Let us not forget that in those days the notion that high levels of unemployment were a social evil still prevailed. A theological review is not the place for detailed discussions of economic theory. I propose to concentrate on the philosophical and theological questions that form the kernel and basis of the theory that emerged victorious from the debates – neo-liberalism. But let us look at one preliminary question first.

Speaking of philosophical questions in economic theories is no longer so strange in economic and philosophical circles, though there are still some who regard it as heresy. But to speak of theological bases and questions in economics is far more polemical. Many theologians completely deny the possibility and make a radical separation between theology and economics. Others reduce the relationship to a simple application of the social teaching of the church to the field of economics, denying the existence of theological questions lying within the economy itself. Meanwhile, and with increasing frequency, we see politicians, economists and other social scientists using expressions such as 'neo-liberal dogma', 'orthodoxy', 'faith in the market" '*laissez-faire* theology', 'necessary sacrifices', and others deriving from theology, in presenting their arguments and analyses.

Some would discount the question by saying that these terms are being used in a purely analogical sense. But their abundance, in authors either favourable or opposed to the present economic order, obliges us to take the matter more seriously. The length of this article precludes numerous quotations, but one has only to read newspapers, reviews or books to find them. Take Paul Ormerod's book *The Death of Economics* as an example: it contains such statements as, 'The economists of the International Monetary Fund and the World Bank preach *salvation* by means of the market to the Third World . . . An intellectual *orthodoxy* arose . . . *The intensity of faith* demonstrated by the majority of economists . . . Many years ago in economic theory the *fundamental belief* was in vogue that the price of a merchandise – be it bananas or people – is determined by the relative levels of supply and demand' (my italics).[2]

'Salvation', 'faith', 'orthodoxy' and other such terms are not new in economics. The basic nucleus of such theological language was already present in Adam Smith. His famous concept of the 'invisible hand' derives from the theological concept of divine providence. This view of the market as a supra-human entity capable, on the basis of individual egoisms competing in the market place, of producing a non-intentional effect of common good, has always been present in the various theories and ideologies of capitalism. But in the 1970s, with the advent of neo-liberalism, it came to assume a specific and more radical form.

The speech given by F. A. von Hayek, the 'pope' of neo-liberalism, when he accepted the Nobel Prize for Economics in 1974, provides a synthesis of the philosophical-theological nucleus that concerns us here. Its title alone is significant: 'The Pretension to Understanding'.[3] Basically, it consists of a re-reading of the myth of the original sin of Adam and Eve. All economic theories develop, in one way or another, consciously or unconsciously, a theology of sin, since they try to explain the causes of evils to be combatted and put forward means of achieving what they consider the (economic) good.

In his acceptance speech Hayek defined the challenge of the economic crisis of the early 1970s as: 'How can we liberate the free world from the serious threat of galloping inflation?'[4] It is important to note that he reduced the crisis to the problem of inflation, discounting unemployment as a serious problem. Having posed the question in these terms, he replied to it by saying that the crisis was brought about by economic policies recommended by the majority of economists, who shared the belief that we could achieve full employment on a permanent basis. This economic theory, inspired by Keynes, presupposes, in Hayek's view, the possibility of understanding all the complex phenomena that make up the market. In other words, the basic evil that originates the harm of galloping inflation and the resulting imbalance and instability of the market – the original sin, in theological terms – is the desire to promote the social good consciously and intentionally, which presupposes the pretension to understand the market.

Against this pretension, Hayek defends the idea that the market is an essentially complex structure. As such, he argues, we cannot understand it fully, and therefore we should not pretend to replace the spontaneous processes of the market with conscious human control through economic and social goals. On the basis of this, he says: 'To act according to the belief that we possess the knowledge and power that enable us to plan the processes of society entirely to our taste, knowledge that in fact we do *not* have, will probably cause us great harm.'[5]

From the correct understanding of the market as a complex system and from the consequent recognition of the impossibility of understanding it fully, he deduces the impossibility of directing it according to our wishes, that is, the impossibility of intentionally achieving full employment or other consciously-set economic goals. This intentional and conscious quest, according to him, will cause us great harm. It is clear that, in the context of his critique of pretensions to absolute understanding of social reality, he cannot state categorically that these desired goods translated into political and economic actions will necessarily cause great harm. So he presents it as a strong possibility.

Harm as a non-intentional effect of an action that seeks the social good comes about, he maintains, through the fact that this action of coercion on other persons or social groups by an authority impedes 'the functioning of those forces of spontaneous disposition through which, without understanding them, man is in fact so fully assisted in the quest for his objective';[6] that is, it impedes the free functioning of the market.

Once social actions planned on the basis of good intentions are seen as generating socio-economic crisis, only two courses are open. One is to take a radically nihilist stance and defend the impossibility of ever having a better world. This type of social theory is, however, frustrating by its nature and doomed to political failure. The other is to believe and hope that the solution to economic and social problems will arrive through the actions of a god or through the non-intentional effects produced by an intrinsically beneficent economic system – that is, the market. As it is impossible to prove empirically that the market system produces only and inevitably social benefits, we have to have faith in it. That is why Milton Friedman, recipient of the Nobel Prize for Economics in 1976, claims that 'underlying most of the arguments against the free market is a lack of faith in freedom as such'.[7]

The alternative to the nihilist position and faith in a transcendentalized market is to take on our human responsibility to work out, democratically, our social goals and to try to put them into effect. This clearly presupposes not only our capacity to understand the dynamic of the market, at least in part, but also the legitimacy of a certain social and legal coercion on sections of society, such as, for example, a progressive tax system to ensure a better distribution of wealth or control over certain types of production or consumption that pose a threat to the environment – ideas abhorrent to neo-liberals.

Neo-liberalism starts from the epistemological principle of the impossibility of fully understanding the way the economy and trading relationships function and comes to the conclusion that the basic evil, or original sin, is the desire to make the benefit they presuppose the object of understanding. Given the impossibility of doing good, the only thing left is the choice to try not to do harm. And the basic harm to be avoided is 'the temptation to do good'. This, incidentally, is the title of a novel written by Peter Drucker, the 'high priest' of business management. In this, a Bishop O'Malley says that the only fault of Zimmerman, the protagonist, 'is to have exercised a little Christian compassion', in that 'he did not resist the temptation to do good'.[8]

This is the reason why unemployment is no longer seen as an economic and social evil to be combatted, and why economic policy has been reduced to the struggle against inflation, so as to maintain confidence in money and in the market. The 'In God we trust' stamped on the dollar shows that trust in money and in the market is as basic as trust in God, since basically the market has been elevated to the status of a god. This is what liberation theologians call the idolatry of the market.

3. Justice and solidarity?

This central core of neo-liberalism, established in a 'probabilist' fashion by Hayek in 1974, has today been raised to the level of dogmatic certainty. It is not by chance that so many economists and sociologists make use of the concept of dogmatism in analysing neo-liberalism and the present dynamic of globalization. Fundamentalism is not only a problem relating to religious groups. The most predominant and perverse fundamentalism today is economic. Social, cultural and historical differences are left out of account when the orthodox prescriptions of the IMF and the World Bank are imposed on undeveloped countries. Social disasters have no effect on belief in the universal validity of their orthodoxy. They claim that increases in poverty and social exclusion are the results not of applying their dogmas, but of not applying them rigorously enough.

When the search for good is considered the basic cause of harm, and when unconcern and cynicism in the face of social problems are seen as the best ethical approach, it is no use preaching social justice and solidarity in the abstract. This is because social justice has been reduced to the efficiency of the market. Efficiency measured by competitiveness in the market is today considered the best criterion for discerning social questions. Therefore, as J. K. Galbraith has shown, one of the main characteristics of our societies is the belief that those who enjoy the riches and benefits brought by the market 'are doing no more than reap their just reward', and 'if good fortune is deserved or if it is a reward for personal merit, there is no plausible justification for any action that may come to prejudice it or inhibit it – that will come to reduce what is or could be enjoyed'.[9] Which means that the poor and unemployed must suffer the 'just deserts' of their own incompetence. This perverse culture is the most dominant version of the theology of retribution in our time.

Solidarity, a concept so dear to Christianity and so important in our days, has not been immune to this inversion either. The speech given by Michel Camdessus, the director general of the IMF, to participants in the National Congress of the CFPC, for owners and directors of Christian firms, in Lille, shows this inversion clearly. He said: 'You are men of the market and of business, seeking efficiency for the sake of solidarity. The International Monetary Fund was set up for international solidarity in the service of countries in crisis which try to make their economies more efficient. The search for efficiency is in and through the market, and you and I both know how related efficiency and solidarity finally are: we stand on the same ground.'[10]

The statement that the IMF is in the service of solidarity will strike many people as being as strange as the headline on celebration at the start of this article. Anyone with even minimal experience of the social consequences of the forced implementation of IMF programmes in the countries of the Third and Fourth Worlds will be indignant at such a claim. But, beyond indignation, we need to understand the logic behind such a statement.

The key lies in the relationship between efficiency in and through the market and solidarity. For the dominant economic school of thought, it is possible to exercise solidarity with the poor only through economic growth. This is because this school identifies quality of life with the quantity of economic goods provided by the Gross National Product. This is seen as the only way of obtaining this growth and, therefore, of exercising solidarity and increasing economic efficiency through free competition in the market. Outside the market there is no salvation!

Once this dogma is adopted *a priori*, one can only practise solidarity by denying solidarity – by, that is, imposing programmes of economic adjustment which increase unemployment, social inequality and other social problems in the name of increased market efficiency. When the IMF is presented as an agent promoting solidarity, all those groups which work in solidarity with the poor, fighting for greater social justice and so upholding alternative political and economic policies, are seen as bringing about the crisis and, therefore, fomenting evil. They are those who fall into the 'temptation to do good'.

According to this school of thought, social inequality is no longer considered a social evil. On the contrary, it is seen as something inevitable, just and beneficent. Inevitable, because it is the necessary outcome of the only possible economic system, the market system. Just, because it is the fruit of the wise distribution of wealth by the market, according to the efficiency of each individual. And beneficent, because it is social inequality that drives people into competition, the engine of economic growth, and is the proof that the state is not intervening in the economy.

4. Solidarity and critique of idolatry

If we fail to unmask this inversion brought about by the market mentality, our works and actions in favour of social justice and solidarity run a serious risk of falling into a void or, worse still, of being interpreted in the sense given them by the neo-liberals. This unmasking has to be done through the process of theological critique of market idolatry. It is this idolizing, this transcendentalizing of the market, which makes the inversion of good and evil possible and legitimate, and which presents the sufferings and deaths of human beings and the destruction of nature as sacrifices necessary for salvation.

In this struggle it is vital for us to re-establish the true meaning of good and evil, of solidarity and cynicism. This is a challenge that does not stop in the economic and ethical fields, but reaches to the heart of theologies and religions. When we talk of the economy today, we are talking of faith, beliefs, dogmas, sacrifices, transcendentalized systems, gods and anthropologies. The problem of evil in the market is, basically, a problem of the theology of sin, of original sin. Sin, grace, salvation . . . are themes that need reflection by theologians within the complexity of contemporary economies and societies.

In the struggle for greater social justice and solidarity, we must take care not to fall into the temptation of trying to build a perfect society, one with no evil in interpersonal and societal relationships, a society in which it is possible to foresee, control, and avoid everything we consider harmful and in which people are completely unselfish and generous. This, besides being epistemologically impossible, would be a negation of our human condition. Criticizing the idolatry of the market does not mean absolute denial of the market or of trading relations as such. As Hugo Assmann says: 'Among undeniable facts, in the field of human interactions in complex societies, is the existence and working of dynamic, partially self-regulating systems in what concerns human behaviour. In the economy, this fact has a name . . . the market.'[11] In other words, our critique of the inversion born of absolutization of the market has to be complemented with a critical but positive acceptance of the market, coupled with a strong emphasis on goals of solidarity.

However well we are able to construct an alternative society – and we have to make the maximum effort to do so – economic and social problems will not disappear completely. One of the reasons for this is that the sum total of human desires will always be greater than existing or future economic goods, so generating conflicts, envies and other evils. Besides this, there is a multiplicity of human, social, and natural factors outside our control.

This being the case, we have to struggle, in the political field and in civil society, to make solidarity take root as a social value. And this is not an easy task, since solidarity is not the only impulse moving human beings; it is rather the fruit of conversion, which is often a very difficult personal process. Without the establishment of solidarity as an objective social norm and value, the suffering of the poor will be seen not as a social evil, but only as a necessary sacrifice or debt due to the sin of economic inefficiency. What makes a correct perception of economic-social evil possible, looking beyond the inversions of the market system, is not only a correct understanding of economic theory but, and most basically, openness to others, solidarity with those who are suffering.

Translated by Paul Burns

Notes

1. *O Estado de Sao Paulo*, 8 February 1997.
2. P. Ormerod, *The Death of Economics*, London 1994.
3. F. A. von Hayek, 'The Pretension to Understanding' (published in Portuguese in *Humanidades* 5, 1983, 47–54).
4. Ibid., 47.
5. Ibid., 54.
6. Ibid.
7. M. Friedman, *Capitalism and Freedom*, 1962.
8. P. Drucker, *The Temptation to Do Good*, 1984.
9. J. K. Galbraith, *The Culture of Contentment*, 1992.
10. M. Camdessus, 'Marché-Royaume: la double appartenance', *Documents Episcopat, Bulletin du Secrétariat de la Conférence des Evêques de France* 12, 1992, 1.
11. H. Assman, *Metáforas novas para reencantar a educaçao*, 1996, 64.

11 · Biblical/Theological Interpretation

'Neither he nor his parents have sinned . . .' Guilt and Exclusion
Hermann Häring

The untouchables and those with a special mark exist in all cultures and play a role in all religions. They are those who feel threatened by a society, who symbolize God's punishment and thus God's justice. Michel Foucauld showed us more than thirty years ago, in his classic investigation of madness in Western culture, how people in Europe dealt with leprosy, later with venereal diseases, and finally with madness.[1] First of all I shall investigate this history and the present situation (I). Then I shall indicate some aspects which make possible a new religious way of dealing with the modern plagues (II).

I. The two faces of Western culture

1. From religious dignity to social control

European culture has two faces: it has been a culture shaped by solidarity and at the same time by anxiety. Of course it accepted its sick people and those marked out by madness. They were under God's special protection, just as Cain already received a sign 'that no one who came upon him should kill him' (Gen. 4.15), or like the leper Lazarus, who at his death was carried by angels into Abraham's bosom (Luke 16.22). Thus in the fifteenth century lepers were still being told that God did not despise them for their sickness and that he did not keep them far from his community.[2] Those who had been smitten by sickness became in a special way witnesses to the suffering that Christ had taken upon himself for the salvation of the whole world. So anyone who excluded from society those who bore a mark was excluding Christ himself. At the same time Christ appears as the fool scorned by his tormentors, whose fate finally makes us ask – right down into contemporary literature, 'Where is real madness to be sought in society?' Thus at the beginning of modernity, plague victims and the mad were still given their own religious dignity. Since the Middle Ages they have been cared for in their own institutions in the name of the Holy, the healing, Spirit.[3] Even now, this voice of solidarity, often with a Christian motivation, has not fallen silent.

However, those who bore a mark have paid a high price for this protection: they have had to succumb to their fate and endure it in patience. European culture, like all cultures, also reacted with anxiety. Those with a mark bore on their body a sign of God's unfathomable nature and the abysses of death. The fear of infection was merely a subsidiary motive for excluding them from society, which supplemented the religious motive.[4] Those hurt in body or spirit could no longer attest God's goodness. Lepers, the syphilitic and the mentally ill were imprisoned in special houses, the latter often driven away or banished on to ships. According to Catholic canon law, as late as 1983 offensive physical malformations were still a bar to receiving priestly orders. The pattern of the leper, who is in fact removed from the community of his people and has to look on it from afar (Luke 17.21), has continued in many ways. This elementary reaction of repudiation and exclusion, further intensified by the great plague epidemics in the Middle Ages, this lively fear of all that is ugly, unquestionably has archaic roots and has hardly been tamed even in the Christian sphere. The balance between exclusion and solidarity therefore always remains uneven and extremely fragile.

In the course of the Enlightenment the pattern of religious dignity was imperceptibly changed into a pattern of public control. Medical science increased, as did the concern for an ordered state. Gradually the conviction became established that we could suppress the great plagues of humanity and are not handed over to any universal human fate. The deviations could be controlled, rationally, technically or medically. Now solidarity was expressed in therapeutic measures. Anxiety became a concern about infection and the disturbance of public order. Measures against plagues took the place of exorcism and public vows. However, there was a further serious change. The holy fear of those who had been smitten might have been repressed, but a moral component now took its place. The more the world was understood as a web of cause and effect, the more people also began to explain sickness and wars from unilinear causes. Granted, this explanation, too, went back to old biblical patterns: Job already resisted the thesis that all suffering must be the result of guilt. However, there was a strong collective notion of this connection between suffering and guilt until well into the Middle Ages. It had above all concerned transgressions of communities, peoples or the whole of humankind, with a mythical origin in the sin of Adam. But now the guilt of the individual stood at the centre; the one who was tormented automatically and directly became a transgressor. Thus a comprehensive process of fixing guilt began from the thirteenth century on, and reached its climax in the nineteenth century.[5] Beyond question, those who bore a mark were now thrown back more mercilessly on themselves than they had been before. Thus the new rationalized syndrome of guilt again attaches itself to those who are to be lamented as the victims of public catastrophes.

2. *The new situation: real apocalyptic*

The late consequences of this development have yet to be overcome, but they have been heavily undermined: for at the latest since the 1960s Christian theology has reacted strongly to this fixation on punishment and guilt. A number of reasons might be mentioned for this. The main reason is the development in the world situation. The ideology of modernity has lost its power of conviction. The new, real and possible catastrophes for humankind can no longer be coped with by the old theological thought-patterns. Here are four components which are stamped by the new catastrophes of humankind: globality, the feasibility and apocalyptic urgency of catastrophes, and the intensified helplessness of the victims.

• *Globality*: the great catastrophes of humankind have attained world-wide dimensions (environmental pollution, nuclear accidents, the gulf between North and South). The weal and woe of the whole of humankind is at risk in them, for any disaster which is brought about anywhere in the world at some time rebounds on those who have caused it. With a few narrowly defined exceptions (for which there are medical grounds), there is therefore no longer any point in excluding concerned groups and thus banishing disaster. The old mechanisms of exclusion arise out of an archaic principle, but this principle is blind and useless for our time, since the new catastrophes for the world and humankind no longer follow the rule '*Sauve qui peut*', but the merciless principle of 'all or nothing'. These are primarily disasters which no longer differentiate between the guilty and the innocent, but whose victims we all become. With or without the ozone layer the sun shines on the evil and the good; Chernobyl irradiated the just and the unjust (Matt. 5.45). Thus solidarity becomes a rationally compelling means of one's own salvation.

• *Feasibility*: the decisive catastrophes for humankind at the present time (epidemics, famine, periods of drought, a lack of water) no longer break upon us unexpectedly; in part they can be foreseen, and in part it is feasible to bring them about. They can be brought on by global, political and technological influences; they can at least be limited, if not prevented altogether, by co-ordinated action world-wide. So the question about their causes and causers has intensified enormously, and it can also be answered in more concrete terms than before. Here we are no longer pointed towards universal postulates which can be misused politically and socially, which make the catastrophes that come about understandable only after the event. Rather, we can begin with an empirical quest for causes and causers; at the same time this makes it possible to develop strategies for avoiding further catastrophes. It is beyond dispute that such a quest can lead to very complex results. But the new way of identifying guilt, whether technological, political or ideological, can make the discussion far more objective and overcome the abstract fixation of guilt and the consequent delusion of innocence in Western culture. As a result of the quest for objectifiable causes, the deeper question of avoidable guilt can at the same time be put more precisely and objectively. This process of objectification is of enormous significance for the theological question of guilt and forgiveness.

• *Apocalyptic urgency*: the new catastrophes for humankind (war, nuclear weapons, genocide, the emissions of poisons and carbon oxides) can lead to global catastrophes as a result of the technological possibilities of the present and the world-wide interconnection between them.

1. In contrast to former eras, the apocalypse is no longer the result of an excited imagination which envisages the impossible and deliberately goes beyond the present scene. Today it is also proving to be technically possible, something that we are playing through as tomorrow's reality. The danger projected becomes extrapolated reality. Here more use of the senses is needed, since whereas the traditional apocalyptic even imagined the impossible, as a result of a theology which has lost the dimension of the senses we can no longer imagine what is possible.[6] So it is time to come to grips with the apocalyptic fantasy, instead of paying homage to a spiritualized eschatology.

2. Even more threatening is the fact that we human beings are adapting ourselves in technologized societies: in other words, changing mentally and in our attitudes. As can in fact be demonstrated, industrialized societies fall victim to the dynamics of their own technology in a way which can no longer be directed.[7] One might think, for example, of the fascination of the car and the aeroplane and technologized households, of the influences of modern genetics and medicine, of the consequences of modern communications and the leisure industry. Together with these often long-term and unforeseeable influences of technical and social innovations,[8] time is becoming a pressing factor. Therefore an open gaze,

sharpened by concern and empathy, must replace the current calculation of guilt and atonement.[9] The fixation on guilt in the Western world has distorted people's view of the possible need of the world; therefore a rethink is of vital importance.

- *The helplessness of the victims*: certainly the victims of catastrophes were helpless at all times. They were exposed to marginalization, pain and death. But in sickness, flooding and famines, as a rule help was also near; today the great catastrophes are usually embedded in a social or political environment of accentuated helplessness. Those concerned are primarily people or groups from whom possible help has been withheld or is made dependent on political conditions: those without possessions; the illiterate; those who are socially, culturally or ethnically marginalized; aliens; the old; mothers or children. As a rule they are incapable of helping themselves. Superficially they often seem to bring disaster upon themselves. Soil is then over-exploited and forests are cut down; seed-corn is eaten and the last reserves of water are wasted; there is little trace of any hygienic measures. However, in many cases this analysis is deceptive, for first of all the poor and dependent are manipulated politically, economically or psychologically as elements in greater mechanisms. So they get caught up in hopeless long-term entanglements and can no longer help themselves. Thus it would be cynical still to interpret the situation of those involved as God's punishment and as a result to cement this situation further; those to be punished would be the perpetrators, the social centres of power, knowledge and capital. On the contrary, help can only come by strengthening the situation of the victims and making it the starting point for new reflections.

II. Towards a new attitude

The conclusions drawn from this by rational theological reflection are therefore clear: traditional religious reactions like exclusion and reference to a universal fate, the fixation of those concerned on sin and guilt, and a superficial optimism for the future, are inappropriate. Only solidarity, an analysis of the causes, direct action, and partisan support of the poor can help further. But that does not conclude the analysis. For the question remains why religious people in particular still react irrationally in all cultures: with exclusion, an assignation of guilt, and the ideas of atonement and appropriate punishment. There are several reasons for this, including assimilation of the vital terror and misuse of it to bring relief to themselves. Only those who are clear about this difficulty can credibly argue for a new form of behaviour.

1. *Why exclusion and repression?*

• *Religious terror*: the great catastrophes of humankind do not present themselves to us as analytical problems but as a vital threat to our future. They do not arouse our intellectual or technological curiosity, but an immediate terror which does not allow any postponement, any detached behaviour, any time-consuming mediation of interpretation. That is also true of the present-day catastrophes of humankind. They throw us back on our helplessness and limitations. For life and death we are delivered over to nature, our bodies and one another. The result is an anxiety about existence and a loss of identity, a loss of orientation, and naked egotism. Thus tremendous abysses appear, the limits to all meaning, the fragility of any future. The great world catastrophes show the cosmos, life and community no longer as protective power but as bottomless demonism, as contempt for a naive belief in God. Thus it is evident that the situation cannot be coped with by idealistic humane answers; situations have to be worked through existentially.

Therefore the modern plagues are once again of the highest religious importance, for in them it becomes clear how we are delivered over to the deadly forces of nature and the inherent destructiveness of society. Now that is the central theme of religion.[10] Certainly physical, psychological or social violence and destruction are conjured up and perpetrated by human beings. But after a certain point we can no longer direct them. The religious reaction to the plagues is therefore always a new collective terror and shared dismay. It issues in lamentation, cries and prayers. But religious action does not stop here; for this dismay both creates all solidarity and at the same time undermines it. Solidarity has the last word and at the same time does not go far enough. But those involved are thrown directly into the situation of which they are victims and reinforce it subjectively by their reaction. At this point we need to see what a religion can achieve and what it cannot: religion does not provide any correct answers (this is especially a misunderstanding of modern theology), but seeks to withstand situations at their utmost limits and to assimilate them. In view of the apocalyptic urgency, religions and a vital religious feeling are always playing with fire, with the frontier between rescue and disaster, with the risk of violence or reconciliation. They must take that risk. They therefore provide a dynamic for the tension between solidarity and anxiety, and are thus always in danger of lapsing into archaic reactions: into the rejection of the other and the one who poses a threat, into the exclusion and stigmatization of the victims. But religion can overcome only what it allows and takes seriously. Defensive reactions and guilty feelings are thus not the sign of a false religion but of an immature religion, a form of religious feeling which has not come into its own.

• *Misuse for one's own relief*: a second reason is more suspect. It is true and, as I have demonstrated, understandable that the thought-pattern of exclusion, victim and divine punishment can also be found in the Bible – as in other cultures.[11] One need only think of Sodom and Gomorrah, of Jonah's descent into the waves, or of the figure of the scapegoat or the flood. By the standards of a contemporary humanity, is not the criticism of such thought-patterns obvious? Now a careful investigation of the Bible could show how intensively such a way of thinking is already criticized there: 'Neither he nor his parents have sinned, but that the works of God might be made manifest in him' (John 9.3), says Jesus unmistakably about the fate of the blind man. He thus says that fellowship, forgiveness and the acceptance of the other are appropriate. If it is a matter of guilt, then we are all entangled in it. That is well known not only in religious circles, but also in all those circles which have some intellectual life. Nevertheless, the societies which are dominant today attempt to ward off catastrophes literally and against all reason, or to exploit them for their own advantage. Fights over distribution, self-preservation and a dismantling of solidarity rather than the call for divine justice are the reasons why we have to keep hearing that the poor are to blame for their own situation, why those sick with AIDS are slandered and street children are shot, why the homeless are despised and the dirty are pushed even deeper into the dirt, why starving refugees are forced even deeper into the jungle. As Eric Fromm remarks, a defence against all uncontrolled and vulnerable life is the hallmark of a 'modern' life orientated on productivity.[12] Fromm calls modern technological societies necrophilic, because they shut themselves off from life and its internal threats. Precisely because of these rationalizations of guilt, the modern plagues seem like the physical and social embodiment of the delusions of those societies which should be concerned with healing them.

2. Towards a new apocalyptic spirituality

So how should religions deal with the new catastrophes? As I have already said, no religion, not even Christian faith, offers an answer to this question. Even discipleship of Jesus is not a recipe, but a painfully creative process. Certainly perspectives can be demonstrated which lead to a new and fruitful way of dealing with our human catastrophes. I shall sum up this way with the words nearness, relationship, responsibility and the option for the victims.

- *Nearness*: catastrophes of humankind are of the utmost anthropological significance for religions and religious feelings. Initially religions do not distance themselves from catastrophes and do not suppress the possibility of catastrophes, but set human beings directly in this world and its life-threatening dangers. Contact with catastrophes, feeling them and enduring them, sharpens the experience of nearness. Victims are delivered over helpless to the torturer or murderer, the quaking earth, fire, and also hunger or Ebola. Tomorrow we can be killed or crushed, choked within ten minutes. Evidently we must first fit into these situations of helplessness and dependence on superhuman powers. So first of all we have to learn that chaos and death slumber in everything; they enter us in contact with the world. So anxiety is part of life. The consistent acceptance of this our life is the only way of overcoming the tendencies towards segregation, constant purification and exculpation.
- *Relationship*: to this is directly attached a second, fundamentally religious experience of life. We live not only as part of reality, but also in relation to it. So there is not only the polarity of contact and separation, of destruction and flight, but also that of reflection and contrast, of affirmation and negation. Between human beings and reality there is a manifold net of relationships: this makes the world situation our own situation. In it we recognize our hopes and our longings, our selves and our love. Therefore the catastrophes of humankind do not speak a neutral language, but also the language of our own death. Evidently there is a great web of disaster in humankind from which even those who have escaped it once again need to be rescued. Of course this network of relationship involves trust or protest, surrender or resistance. But much more fundamentally it calls for watchfulness of the spirit, for a sensitivity to the reality which we are and which at the same time surrounds us, a sensitivity which is ready to hear. This sensitivity is of the utmost importance for dealing with catastrophes in a humane way, since it alone creates openness, detachment and a fundamental freedom. Without it religion and religious awareness are restricted to techniques of deterrence and magic; the experience of our common fate becomes a fixation on a shared guilt,[13] with the fear of hell and damnation. This restriction in particular opens the way to uncontrolled and inhuman projections. That also makes a hesitation to offer clear answers more important here, along with a sensitivity to the interconnections of disaster which escape immediate perception.
- *Responsibility*: the same goes for the search for culprits and guilt. Certainly individuals and groups must be specifically called to account for what they have done. The discovery of this perspective in Jewish and European culture is one of the greatest pieces of progress, which has been

taken over uncurtailed by the monotheistic religions. But at the latest after the time of Augustine, the category of imputable guilt was universalized into a general guilt on the part of humankind[14] and thus made inoperable. This theory stills any protest and even any empirical enquiry into shares in guilt and suffering.

Now Hans Küng has proposed a pragmatic approach in his *Global Responsibility*. This is a readiness to discuss global interconnections critically,[15] to make sober analyses and to measure the threats to the world by the traditions of the great religions. Another task of the religions and their theologies is collaboration in a new global awareness. This awareness must perceive the world in its internal world-wide connections, not only of salvation but also of disaster. Here there is a need to exercise not only a sensitivity to the reality which surrounds us but also a readiness to take responsibility for the long-term future of the world, regardless of concrete guilt. That is not a past disaster but – directed towards the future – a guilt which human beings can only atone for together and in solidarity.

• *Option for the victims*: nevertheless, this global approach asks too much of theology and faith. Can we really find the universal world solution? In this plural world do we not irrevocably remain imprisoned, each in his or her own cultural perspectives and interests? Certainly a universal programme of humanity is no help unless it contains clear perspectives which reduce the excessive complexity of the question. Here I am referring to a biblically Christian memory which has been brought to the centre again in liberation theology. René Girard already investigated the question whether the biblical message offers a specific approach for overcoming disaster. His answer was that the Bible regards questions of suffering and injustice, violence and death, not from the perspective of the victors but from the perspectives of the defeated. That is true of many central passages of Holy Scripture.

It is quite certainly true of the memory of the life of Jesus of Nazareth, whom God chose as his Son precisely at the moment of the deepest abandonment. Thus Christian faith lives from the central experience that God is to be found on the side of the defeated. So the guideline for a Christian interpretation of the world is the fate of the defeated. This must also be the guideline for our dealings with the new catastrophes of the world and humankind. However, this has practical consequences. The exclusion of the victim, the search for scapegoats and the projection of divine judgments of damnation will be forbidden us in the future. Now it is high time to help and heal, for 'the night will come in which no one can work' (John 9.3f.).

Translated by John Bowden

Notes

1. M. Foucault, *Madness and Civilization* (1961), London 1967.
2. There is more in ibid., ch. 1, 'Ship of Fools'. One might think of the Isenheim altar, which even now exercises a great fascination on artists; here one might think of Otto Dix or Jasper Johns.
3. As the metaphor of evil shows, anxiety about pollution and infection always plays a great role. In Greek mythology Thebes is smitten with plague because of the crime of Oedipus. Augustine explains the universality of 'original sin' among other things as the result of a universal infection.
4. The healing and caring mentality of this worship of the Holy Spirit is expressed very emphatically in the hymn 'Veni Creator Spiritus'.
5. J. Delumeau, *Le péché et la peur. La culpabilisation en Occident (Xllle–XVIIIe siècles)*, Paris 1983.
6. G. Anders, *Die Antiquiertheit des Menschen* (2 vols), Munich 1987.
7. E. Martens, *Zwischen Gut und Böse. Elementare Fragen angewandter Philosophie*, Stuttgart 1997, 180–99, on 'How is peace possible?'
8. G. Altner, *Naturvergessenheit. Grundlagen einer umfassenden Bioethik*, Darmstadt 1991.
9. H. Häring, 'De redding komt alleen van God: Het laatste oordeel bezien vanuit de apokalyptiek', *Tijdschrift voor Theologie* 33, 1993, 348–70; id., '"Uitschreeuwen wat er gaande is": Over de relevantie van eschatologie en apokalyptiek', *Tijdschrift voor Theologie* 36, 1996, 246–69.
10. R. Girard, *Violence and the Sacred*, Baltimore 1979.
11. The multiple sequence of world catastrophes in the Hopi myths, which is also caused by human injustice, is interesting; cf. F. Waters, *Book of the Hopi*, New York 1963.
12. E. Fromm, *The Anatomy of Human Destructiveness*, New York 1973.
13. The following remarks are based on P. Ricoeur, *The Symbolism of Evil* (1960), Boston 1969, which has now become a classic, especially Part 1.
14. P. Ricoeur, 'Le "péché originel": Etude de signification', *Eglise et théoIogie, Bulletin trimestriel de la faculté de Theologie protestante de Paris* 23, 1960, 11–30; H. Hanno, *Macht des Bosen, Das Erbe Augustins*, Gütersloh 1979, 181–267.
15. H. Küng, *Global Responsibility*, London and New York 1991; id., *A Global Ethic for Global Politics and Global Economics*, London 1997.

Plagues in the Bible
Exodus and Apocalypse

Pablo Richard

Introduction

Plagues, catastrophes and calamities have always been an uncontrollable and incomprehensible subject, and one that has been manipulated to spread terror and destruction. And yet the two books of the Bible, Exodus and the Apocalypse (or Book of Revelation), in which the subject of plagues is treated, first historically and then cosmologically, are precisely the books with the most powerful message of liberation and hope for the people of God and for the early Christian communities. In these books plagues always have a positive meaning for the people of God, especially for the poor and oppressed.

Both texts contain two traditions: in one, plagues are the signs and wonders worked by God himself, to damage the system so as to permit the liberation of the people of God and the building of the kingdom of God on earth; in the other, plagues represent the violence of the system of domination itself, which is eventually turned against it, thereby still, on a positive note, allowing for a stocktaking and a transformation of the situation. The context that gives a positive sense to plagues is always the march of humankind toward the promised land, the construction of the kingdom on earth and the utopia of living in a new earth and new heaven and in the new Jerusalem, which comes down to earth from heaven.

In this article I propose to examine first the meaning of plagues in Exodus and the Apocalypse, so as then to reflect on present-day plagues in the light of the biblical books.

I. Plagues in the book of Exodus

The so-called plagues of Egypt appear in 7.1–13.16.[1] The classical name 'plague' strictly applies only to the tenth, the death of the firstborn. The nine previous plagues are rather presented as 'signs and wonders' (7.3) and can be interpreted as natural phenomena. The water turned to blood (7.14–25) can be explained by the swelling of the river Nile, which brings down red earth; red is interpreted mythologically as blood. The frogs, the gnats (or mosquitoes), the flies, the pestilence that killed the livestock, the festering boils, the hail, the locusts, and the darkness (7.28–10.29) are all possible natural phenomena, but here presented in mythological form and as signs and wonders worked by Yahweh, given excessive and unlikely intensity, and affecting only the Egyptians. Before these nine 'plagues' there is a different prodigy: Moses' staff transformed into a snake (7.10); after the nine comes a tenth, also different in character. This is not a natural phenomenon exaggerated but a genuine plague, wounding the Egyptians directly and mortally, killing all the firstborn of both humans and animals.

What theological meaning do these plagues in Exodus have? The social context of the first nine 'plagues' is the peasant struggles against the city-state, concerning the payment of tribute. It is the response of tribes subjected to the royal house, when oppression reached unbearable limits. These plagues are forceful measures taken by the tribes to defend themselves against the oppressive system. In the book of Exodus they are interpreted theologically as signs and wonders worked by Yahweh, giving him credit in Pharaoh's eyes as the God who liberates the Hebrew tribes. Yahweh damages or strikes the structures of domination, thereby allowing the people of God to go free. These accounts date from the period of exodus, but were later re-worked during the struggle of the Hebrew tribes against the Canaanite kings; and again in the context of the prophets' struggle against the kings of Israel and Judah: Nathan against David, Elias against Ahab; Amos against Jeroboam II; Isaiah against Ahaz, and so on . . .

The tenth plague, the death of the firstborn, has a different theological meaning. The book of Exodus begins with the pitiless exploitation of the Israelites (1.8–14), and its cruellest manifestation – the command to the midwives to kill newborn boy children (1.15–22). Now it is the firstborn of the Egyptians who are wounded to death. The Egyptians, who began by commanding that the Hebrew boys should be killed, end by suffering the death of their own sons. It is the death of the oppressed that leads to the killing of the sons of the oppressors. This is not a sign or wonder from

Yahweh, but the violence of the oppressors themselves turned against them. The signs and wonders of the first nine 'plagues' damage Pharaoh so that he will agree to terms on which to release the Hebrews, but in this tenth there is no negotiation at all: Pharaoh recognizes his utter defeat and agrees to all Moses' demands without any conditions whatsoever (12.31–32). The plague of the death of the Egyptian firstborn is included in the narration of the institution of three rites: Passover, unleavened bread, and redemption of the firstborn (the plague is recounted in 12.29–42, in the ritual context of 12.1–13.16). Here myth is united to rite. The rites serve to perpetuate the myth, and both have a liberating meaning. In the celebration of the rite the people recall how God wounded Egypt and how he protected them with the blood of the Passover lamb.

II. Plagues in the book of the Apocalypse

The classic texts on plagues in the Apocalypse are basically in 8.2–11.19 (the section on the seven trumpets) and 15.5–16.21 (the seven bowls).[2] In the overall structure of the book, these two sections are in strict parallel. Both represent a re-reading of the book of Exodus, no longer in Egypt, but at the heart of the Roman empire at the end of the first century of the Christian era. Looking rapidly at the structure of these sections, we shall see that both begin with a vision of a portent in heaven (8.2–6 and 15.5–16.1); this represents the liturgy of the Christian community, which is suffering from the 'plagues' of the seven trumpets and the seven bowls. The first four trumpets and the first four bowls tell of cosmic plagues, striking the earth, the sea, the rivers and sources of water, and finally the sun (8.7–12 and 16.2–9). The plague of the fifth trumpet is described in more detail: a star fallen from heaven opens the shaft of the bottomless pit, and out come locusts, with the king the angel of the bottomless pit (9.1–11). The plague of the fifth bowl falls on the throne of the beast and plunges its kingdom into darkness (16.10–11). The plague of the sixth trumpet is of the four killer angels from the river Euphrates with their troops of two hundred million cavalry (9.13–21), and the parallel plague of the sixth bowl falls on the same river Euphrates, drying up its waters to allow the kings from the east to pass over (16.12–16). The 'plague' announced by the seventh trumpet is the coming of the kingdom of God (11.15–19), also told in truncated form in the text of the seventh bowl (16.17–21).

What do all these 'plagues' mean? The reply is in the text itself, which merits close reading. In the first place it is important to ask who suffers the plagues, against whom they are directed in history. Before answering this, it is worth noting that the seven bowls have a more specific and historical character than the plagues of the seven trumpets. As the two texts are parallels, we can make a joint interpretation. The first four plagues have a cosmic character: there is the destruction of a third of the earth, of the sea, of the rivers and sources of water, of the sun, the moon, and the stars (8.6–12). There is strong insistence on the destruction being of only a third part, but it is not said what or who makes up this third. In the parallel text of the seven bowls (16.1–9) this ambiguity is resolved, since it is explicitly stated that the first plague, on the earth, consists of 'a foul and painful sore . . . on those who had the mark of the beast and who worshipped its image'. In the second and third bowls, the sea and all the waters are turned to blood, and a little community liturgy is added, in which the reason for the plague is given: 'because they shed the blood of saints and prophets, you have given them blood to drink. It is what they deserve!' The fourth bowl is not so explicit, but those afflicted by this plague 'cursed the name of God . . . and did not repent'. So, to sum up: those who suffer the four cosmic plagues are those who carry the mark of the beast, who kill the saints and prophets, the impious who blaspheme against the name of God. They are clearly the idolaters and killers who belong to the Roman empire.

The plagues of the fifth, sixth and seventh trumpets, with their parallels of the bowls, are historical rather than cosmic in character. There is a redactional pointer in the section on the trumpets that provides a key for interpretation. Referring to the three blasts of the trumpet yet to come, the author says: 'Woe, woe, woe to the inhabitants of the earth . . .!' (8.13). In the Apocalypse, the expression 'inhabitants of the earth' denotes the impious. In the plague of the fifth trumpet (9.1–11) it is explicitly stated that the satanic locusts are told to damage 'only those people who do not have the seal of God on their foreheads'. In the parallel text of the fifth bowl this is said to be poured 'on the throne of the beast' (16.10–11). The plagues of the sixth trumpet and the sixth bowl (9.13–21 and 16.12) have the river Euphrates as their direct object. The plague consists in the river being dried up so as to give free passage to the kings from the east. The Euphrates was the eastern boundary of the empire, holding back the barbarous nations of the east. These nations are represented in the sixth trumpet by the four killer angels and their two hundred million cavalry.

So, to sum up: these two plagues (the fifth and sixth in the parallel sets of text) are clearly aimed at the Roman empire and its followers. What is most notable is that the plague announced by the seventh trumpet (11.15–19) is presented in parallel with those of the fifth and sixth trumpets (the third 'woe' to the 'inhabitants of the earth': see 8.13; 9.12; 11.14). This curious 'plague' is the coming of the kingdom of God: 'The kingdom of the world has become the kingdom of our Lord and of his Messiah' (11.15–19). The coming of the kingdom is indeed a plague for the Roman empire, since the kingdom of God in the Apocalypse comes about historically on the earth. In the parallel text of the seventh bowl, the coming of the kingdom of God is accompanied by the proclamation of a great cataclysm that destroys Rome, called Babylon, the great city (16.17–21).

What, then, is the purpose or object of these plagues? In the cosmic plagues, there is insistence on the destruction of only a third of the cosmos (8.6–12). The destruction is not total: two thirds remain for grace and conversion. Also in the plague of the fifth trumpet, the locusts do not kill the impious but only torture them for five months (9.5–10); clearly, what is sought is not their death but their conversion. There is the observation, repeated several times, that despite suffering these plagues the wicked are not converted from their crimes and idolatries, but curse God (9.20–21; 16.9, 11, 21). The Apocalypse breathes pessimism on this point, since at no point in the seven trumpets and seven bowls is there the slightest indication of the conversion of the idolaters and criminals against whom all the plagues are directed. If all is lost and no one is converted, why then the plagues? In the section on the seven trumpets, the author has introduced, between the sixth and seventh, a long passage devoted to the activity of the prophets: from 10.1 to 11.13 this describes the actions of a powerful angel who comes down from heaven (10.1–7), the calling and prophetic action of John (10.8–11.2), and the activity, passion, death and resurrection of the prophetic church (11.3–13). Curiously, the end of this prophetic section provides the only positive witness in the Apocalypse to the wicked being converted: 'and the rest were terrified and gave glory to the God of heaven' (11.13).

What this means is this: the seven trumpets, with the proclamation of their respective plagues against the Roman empire, are carried out in history at the present time. The author places himself in the middle of this present time, between the sixth and seventh trumpets. When the seventh trumpet sounds, this present time of grace and conversion comes to an end (this is proclaimed by the prophet angel in 10.6–7). The mission of the prophets in this present time is to secure the conversion of the wicked who bear the mark of the beast. The plagues make sense only in the context of this action by the prophets and the prophetic church. The prophets are those who give meaning to the action of God in damaging the structures of evil in this present time before the final judgment. The prophetic passage between the sixth and seventh trumpets has its antithesis in the parallel text between the sixth and seventh bowls (16.13–16). I say 'antithesis' because here we have the anti-prophetic movement: the demonic spirits, who come out of the structures of death to perform signs and seduce the whole world.

III. Exodus and Apocalypse: an overall vision

What is the overall meaning of the plagues in the light of the books of Exodus and the Apocalypse? One fundamental fact is – as we have already seen – that all plagues are always directed against a system of oppression, never against the people of God or the Christian communities. In the book of Exodus the plagues fall on Pharaoh, Pharaoh's house and the Egyptian people in general (the tributary system of production). In the Apocalypse the plagues fall on the Roman empire and its economic, political and religious systems of domination. There is coherence on this point between Exodus and the Apocalypse. The Apocalypse makes a re-reading of Exodus in the context of the Roman empire. The plagues of the Apocalypse are clearly inspired by those of Exodus, and in both cases they have a negative meaning for the system of domination and a positive and liberating meaning for the people of God. In the two books the plagues are expressed in mythical and symbolic terms, but their content and significance are fully historical.

In both Exodus and the Apocalypse I have made a distinction between two specific types of plague: 1. plagues as signs and wonders worked by God, in order to wound the system of domination and allow the People of God to be freed; 2. plagues as the violence of the system, which is then turned against the system itself. In the first case the direct agent of the plagues is God himself (even if the action of the people is implicitly included); in the second case the direct agent is the system of domination (even if it is God who indirectly allows and sometimes provokes the action). In both cases the object struck by the plagues is the system of domination and object benefited is the people of God. There are two paradigmatic texts in the Apocalypse that clearly express these two types of plagues. The first is in the seventh trumpet, 11.15–18:

> Then the seventh angel blew his trumpet, and there were loud
> voices in heaven, saying,
> > 'The kingdom of the world has become the kingdom of
> > > our Lord and of his Messiah,
> > and he will reign for ever and ever.'
> Then the twenty-four elders who sit on their thrones before God
> fell on their faces and worshipped God, singing,

'We give you thanks, Lord God Almighty,
   who are and who were,
for you have taken your great power
   and begun to reign.
The nations raged,
   but your wrath has come,
   and the time for judging the dead,
for rewarding your servants, the prophets
   and saints and all who fear your name,
   both small and great,
   and for destroying those who destroy the earth.'

The second type of plague, the violence of the system turned against itself, is described in the community liturgy which the author of the Apocalypse inserts between the plagues of the second and third bowls, when all the waters are changed into blood, 16.5–7:

And I heard the angel of the waters say,
   'You are just, O Holy One, who are and were,
   for you have judged these things;
   because they shed the blood of saints and prophets,
   you have given them blood to drink.
   It is what they deserve!'
And I heard the altar respond,
   'Yes, O Lord God, the Almighty,
   your judgments are true and just!'

IV. A present-day re-reading of the plagues of Exodus and the Apocalypse

Today we can see the existence of innumerable plagues, catastrophes, calamities; there are cosmic, biological, economic, social, ethnic, psychological, religious plagues. All kinds of interpretation are given. Let us begin with false interpretations of plagues.

The first is 'naturalist' in character: plagues are interpreted as 'natural disasters', necessary, inevitable, uncontrollable. This interpretation generates an attitude of irresponsible indifference.

Another false interpretation is the eschatological-fundamentalist one: plagues and catastrophes are interpreted as signs of the end of the world and the second coming of Christ; the more plagues the better, since the Lord is near; there is no place for fear, since the 'saints' will be saved from the calamities. This fundamentalist approach endows 'believers' with a complacent and even joyful attitude to catastrophes; it also often leads to terrorist behaviour: catastrophes should be provoked directly, so as to hasten the end of the world and the coming of the new world.

Then there are the ideological-political types of false interpretation: everything that does not belong to the logic of the dominant system is held to be and is presented as a plague, as a calamity – oppressed ethnic groups, migrants, unwanted children, street children, rebellious young people, prostitutes, the poor in general; all these are presented as plagues of modern society, impeding its progress and destroying its nature.

Next, there are the perverse religious interpretations: plagues as God's punishment for sins – AIDS would be the paradigmatic case, God's punishment for sexual sins.

Others explain plagues as destiny, brought on by mysterious occult forces or by the devil himself.

All these false interpretations seek to hide the reality of the oppressed, to legitimize domination, and to de-legitimize those who struggle against it.

We have to make a theological and prophetic discernment of plagues in the light of Exodus and the Apocalypse, which implies making it from the poor, from the victims, from the Third World, and from resistance to systems of domination. We must discern plagues with the Spirit in which Exodus and the Apocalypse were written. We need to distinguish in the present-day situation, as we have just done in the biblical analysis, between violence generated by the system, which turns against the system itself (the only plagues that really deserve the name), and the actions of those who resist and struggle against the system (the signs and wonders of the coming of the kingdom of God). In the light of the Bible, plagues are to be seen as always against the system of domination, never against the poor, the communities, or the people of God. Furthermore, plagues have a positive purpose: they seek not destruction but conversion, and the consequent liberation of the poor.

Let us begin by naming – there being no space here for any deeper analysis – the plagues brought on by the system, in the light of those seen in Exodus (the tenth plague) and in the Apocalypse (the first six trumpets and bowls). First, there are the cosmic plagues; here we can situate all the ecological disasters brought on by the system: deforestation, desertification, droughts, floods, disappearance of animal and plant species, pollution of the atmosphere and of rivers and aquifers, holes in the ozone layer, diseases, genetic malformations, widespread sterility. In this context we can re-read the four cosmic plagues of the Apocalypse (the first four trumpets [8.6–12] and the first four bowls [16.1–9]) and discern the present reality of ecological destruction in the light of these texts. This discernment has to be made on the basis of taking stock of, converting, and changing the oppressive actual situation. If only a third of the cosmos is destroyed, two-thirds remain to be converted.

Besides the cosmic plagues or ecological sufferings there are the human plagues: economic, social, ethnic, and political. The economic plagues weighing on the Third World are payment of the external debt, the pressures of the IMF or the World Bank, the absolutization of the market, the destructive aggressiveness of transnational corporations, consumerism. The social plagues are racism, *machismo*, militarism; the plagues unleashed by the exclusion of the majority of the population from the present free-market capitalist system: forced migrations, social fragmentation, family break-up, criminality, drugs, social epidemics (such as cholera, AIDS, tuberculosis, leprosy); not to mention the communications media when they are promoting consumerism; sexism, violence. Furthermore, there are religious plagues: fundamentalist, integralist and fanatical tendencies perverting the churches, religions, and new religious movements compromising with the violence of the system; then again, terrorist and apocalyptic groups manipulating violence against the people themselves. In this context we should re-read the fifth and sixth trumpets of the Apocalypse (9.1–21) and the fifth and sixth bowls (16.10–12) or the tenth plague in Exodus (the death of the firstborn of Egypt: chs.11–13). All these plagues are generated by the system and then turned against the system. Those who have spilt blood drink blood. Demons come out of the pit of the wickedness and irrationality of the system.

One might raise the objection to all the foregoing that the victims of all these plagues are precisely the poor, those victimized and oppressed by the system. This is true when the poor are completely integrated into the system, but it is not true to the degree that the poor and oppressed resist and struggle against the system. It is in this context of resistance and struggle that we discover the meaning of biblical texts that speak of the 'plagues' as 'signs and wonders of Yahweh' (the first nine plagues of Egypt) and of the 'plagues' that irrupt with the coming of the Kingdom of God (the seventh trumpet and seventh bowl of the Apocalypse). All these first nine plagues of Egypt and all the signs of the coming of the kingdom in the Apocalypse are actualized in the acts of resistance and struggle by the poor and oppressed against the system of domination and for the liberation of the people of God. Let us name all these acts of resistance to domination: political and social, cultural, ethical, and spiritual resistance; all spaces opened up to life; all projects promoting life; all alternative liberation movements, whose agents are the excluded, indigenous peoples, women, young persons, ecological warriors. In all these the kingdom of God is coming. They are negative signs for the system, but they are the signs and wonders of God for the poor, proclaiming and bringing in the kingdom of God.

Translated by Paul Burns

Notes

1. My analysis basically follows Jorge Pixley, *On Exodus: A Liberation Perspective*, Maryknoll, NY 1987.
2. For a deeper analysis see Pablo Richard, *Apocalypse, A People's Commentary on the Book of Revelation*, Maryknoll, NY 1995.

Job: 'Even when I cry out "Violence!" I am not answered'

Elsa Tamez

The return of 'plagues' is, at least partly, an effect of the recent displacement of an international movement that had displayed solidarity with the innocents who suffer. This displacement has created a vacuum, making the return of 'plagues' possible. The globalization of the free market, claiming to occupy all possible space in the field of choices leading to an improvement in human life, invades both private and public spheres, floods in our 'house' (our *oikos*, the planet that belongs to us all), and – perhaps without meaning to – fertilizes the soil to receive the returning 'plagues'. Human history in the 1990s is showing what happens when a house is abandoned: rats and cockroaches occupy it immediately it is empty. The weak and defenceless are being overrun by what many people regard as uncontrollable forces.

The movement of solidarity, broken apart by the vagaries of history, even while it looks for new ways of living well under different systems, has not noticed that its removal from the (explicit) place of solidarity with the poor has, unintentionally, left the door open for the plagues to rush in. Many wise observations can be made on this statement, but the evidence of the alarming deterioration in the standard of life of the poor majorities – in the whole world, not just the Third World – is plain to see: their condition is worse than it has been over the past decades. The difference is that now no one is calling aloud for justice, nor would anyone answer if they did.

Let us listen to Job on the garbage heap: 'Even when I cry out "Violence!" I am not answered; I call aloud, but there is no justice' (19.7). But now those excluded from the city are not calling out, or if they are, they are doing so very quietly, as though they know in advance they will not be heard. There they are working on the garbage heap – collecting, breathing, smelling, eating, touching, and asking for garbage. Perhaps they do not call aloud because the passers-by all have 'walkmans' on. It seems that in the world of the destitute they are beginning to live with 'plagues', including those epidemics that had been eliminated, such as measles, tuberculosis and cholera.

Re-reading Job from this perspective today sets us fresh challenges. Even though the garbage heap is the same, only bigger, the way people act is different. There are 'Jobs' not calling out, there are no 'friends' who attack them in defence of God, and the absence of the Almighty is intolerably prolonged.

Silence and cries are subjects I shall tackle in this reflection on Job in the light of the present situation. But I begin with another question.[1]

I. Question

The central question of the book of Job resides in the suffering of the innocent and the reasons for it. The discourses attempt to confirm either the innocence of the one suffering (Job, against the doctrine of temporal retribution) or his culpability (the 'comforters', defending this doctrine). God's discourse accepts Job's innocence but refuses to accept responsibility for atrocities committed against the innocent. On the level of the meaning of the text, the author of the book of Job cannot, or does not want to, give a reason why people suffer unjustly. In the work, all that is stated, in non-analytical language, is that God has plans that cannot be understood by human beings and that at the end of the day God controls chaos too (chs. 38–41). On the level of the underlying story, the readers know that Job is suffering because the character called Satan and the character called God make a wager on the relationship between God and Job (Prologue). Satan wagers that Job's relationship to God is self-interested and utilitarian: if Job has integrity, it is because God has blessed him with riches and good health. Satan moves within the framework of a market theology. God wagers on a blameless and disinterested relationship; that is, Job serves God 'for nothing'.[2] Thieves, thunderbolts, murderers, hurricanes and finally diseases are used to describe the (secondary) causes of Job's absolute misfortune (1.13–19). Both in the argument of the text and on the level of the background story Job suffers unjustly: in the first for unexplained reasons, in the second on account of the wager. It is made clear that Satan is the engine that produces the spark that causes the suffering of the innocent.

God wins the wager. Job is restored; his experience of suffering as one of the destitute leads him to understand the world in its sadness and misery, and leads him to know a new face of God. Perhaps it has taught him to live with a God at once distant and close.

At the time the book of Job was written, there was possibly no understanding of structural sin (*hamartia*) as Paul conceives it in Romans. There was a greater consciousness that individual transgressions by the wicked caused the suffering of the innocent. God would punish the evil as they deserved and revindicate the victims. If this theology were clear, there would be a certain tranquillity in the world. But it is not. Job is just and innocent and suffers arbitrarily. For Eliphaz, Bildad and Zophar, Job is unjust since he experiences in his flesh what happens to the wicked according to the doctrine of retribution.

Today we have a greater understanding of structural sin, which is engineered by human beings. We see its characteristics more clearly: it is that system whose logic, inspired by profit, causes havoc on all levels of human life and habitat. It is a systemic sin that contaminates relationships between people, making them all accomplices in it. Today, although some individual cases invite us to reflect on undeserved suffering and remain a mystery, we more or less know why most people suffer unjustly and we know that many of our 'plagues' are social constructs. So the question needs to be re-phrased. If we now know, at least partly, why the innocent suffer, if we believe they are not primarily the guilty ones, if we know where they are and something of their misfortune, what we then need to do is to ask ourselves what is or should be our attitude to this suffering of the innocent today, when it seems there are no cries demanding justice nor ears to hear such demands. The rest of this article seeks to extract some pointers from the book of Job to help us recall the importance of the claims of the innocent and reflect on silences and cries.

II. Silences

The book of Job contains various silences, some of deep communion, some yearning, some devastating.

The first and most intense lasts seven days and seven nights. Three friends, Eliphaz, Bildad, and Zophar, each 'set out from his home' and 'met together to go and comfort and console him' (2.11). The narrator tells that when they saw Job from a distance, 'they raised their voices and wept aloud; they tore their robes and threw dust in the air upon their heads. They sat with him on the ground seven days and seven nights, and no one spoke a word to him, for they saw that his suffering was very great' (2.12–13).

Silence is spent in the space of the sufferer. The text says that the friends each set out from his home and came to see Job. They stay in Job's new home, the garbage heap, where Job 'sat among the ashes' (2.8). Arrived there, they are horrified to see his revolting body. Any word spoken is useless at such a time.

Silence is the new wisdom. This is the silence of solidarity that brings souls, tears, and the beating of hearts together in harmony. The only dissonant note is the rasping of the potsherd with which Job scrapes his sores (2.8).

The wisdom of silence is later proclaimed by Job (13.5), but it is not repeated, since discourses devised with wisdom take up the entire scene for the whole of the rest of the book. These complicate the relations of friendship and remove solidarity. Reasoning in a search for the causes of suffering is not the greatest wisdom at such a time. This is compassion, moved by the five senses of the human body. These see, hear, smell, touch, and feel their own tears. They bring a silence of solidarity, intense and moving, which humanizes people and brings them into communion. Being moved by the misfortune of others implies recognizing others as human beings and equally implies humanizing oneself. It is a process of mutual humanization.

There is another type of silence, different and also necessary. These are silences united to the mind and hearing of the listener, silences that instruct. Job several times asks his friends, the wise men, to keep quiet and listen: 'Listen carefully to my words, and let this be your consolation. Bear with me, and I will speak' (21.2). The friends talk and talk and are unable to listen to arguments that go against tradition. The reality of the suffering of the innocent cannot destroy their beliefs. They prefer to defend their mental constructs, thinking they are defending God, to listening to a dissonant voice speaking out of real experience. Job says to them: 'If you would only keep silent, that would be your wisdom! Hear now my reasoning, and listen to the pleadings of my lips (13.5–6) . . . Your maxims are proverbs of ashes, your defences are defences of clay (13.12) . . . Listen carefully to my words, and let my declaration be in your ears' (13.17). Job is also prepared to keep silent so as to listen to new arguments explaining the injustice to him: he asks to be taught and says he will be silent to gain understanding (6.24). These are active silences in a listening attitude, which can serve to change views and attitudes.

Job feels that no one is listening to him: 'Oh, that I had one to hear me!', he cries in 31.35. The words of God, following those of Elihu, will show that God is listening to him.

Not all silences, however, are wise. There are silences that kill. Job feels obliged, out of justice and dignity, to break his silence and defend himself against accusations that it his fault that he finds himself in this sub-human situation. He argues with his friends and with God. Drawing on facts from his own experience, organized into rational countervailing speeches, he insists on the injustice that has been committed. He deals with matters of life and death. If Job does not denounce the unjust order under which the innocent suffer, this will impose itself as being logical, and its irrationality will be masked as reasonable. To keep silent is to die: 'Who is there that will contend with me? For then I would be silent and die' (13.19; Schöckel reads, 'For to be silent now would be to die').[3] To his friends he confesses that he is playing for the ultimate stakes: 'Let me have silence, and I will speak, and let come on me what may' (13.13ff). This was the way he had behaved, even before falling into misfortune (31.34).

God keeps silence, and this silence unleashes Job's cries.

III. Cries

After the intense silence shared for seven days and seven nights has become unbearable, the work changes the rhythm of its general tone. Job's cries and those of his friends break the silence, and a chorus of cries crowned with concrete and abstract arguments takes over the atmosphere on the garbage heap. Twenty speeches are made, ten by Job, nine by the friends (three each), and one by the young man Elihu. In the end, the words and arguments run out: the cries are left with no answer. God – inevitably – will have to add his voice.

Job's cry calls out for justice; it is uttered with force, together with anger and anguish. It is a cry that its author cannot control. Job cries out vehemently, cursing the day he was born (3.1–3), demanding to be heard, proving his innocence, combatting, with arguments drawn from daily life, the falsity of the doctrine of retribution. One can almost say that those reading or watching the drama see, hear, and feel the tragedy.

Job, on getting no reply to his denunciations, turns them against God. The wise friends cannot allow such irreverence.[4] With their traditional arguments, they try to stifle the cries of the sufferer. Cries against cries, one the innocence of the just, others trying to prove him guilty.

In the course of the speeches, Job seems not to be seeking compensation; what he wants is to recover his dignity as a human being. In effect, what is most admirable about Job is not that he refused to curse God, but the fact that he never lost his dignity as a human being. More – he grows in this dignity through the process of denunciation and self-defence: 'Here is my signature! Let the Almighty answer me! Oh, that I had the indictment written by my adversary! Surely I would carry it on my shoulder; I would bind it on me like a crown; I would give him an account of all my steps; like a prince I would approach him' (31.35–37). This is the note on which Job ends his final speech.

Job's cries are those that save, for 'to be silent now would be to die' (13.19). But the cries of the others are useless cries. They discourse outside the actual context, which demonstrates injustices. They defend the Almighty with statements divorced from daily reality, condemning both the just man and themselves. Like Satan, the friends turn into accusers, without meaning to. Job declares: 'I have heard many such things; miserable comforters are you all. Have windy words no limit? Or what provokes you that you keep on talking? I also could talk as you do, if you were in my place; I could join words together against you, and shake my head at you. I could encourage you with my mouth, and the solace of my lips would assuage your pain' (16.2–5).

At times inopportune speeches become so hard they strike like stones. This is how Job feels them, as he asks why his friends torment him and break him in pieces (19.2). In this cul-de-sac, one thing is clear: neither silences nor cries alleviate the suffering of the innocent. Job experiences this in his own flesh: 'If I speak, my pain is not assuaged, and if I forbear, how much of it leaves me?' (16.6).

The literary construction of the book forces God to break his silence, come down to the garbage heap, and add his voice. God, having been called into question, has the right to cry out in response. God shows himself in his own way, re-situating the questions and broadening the visions. God does not accuse Job, as Satan, the friends and Elihu have done. The appearance of God's cry makes it possible for Job to raise himself from the garbage heap, to affirm his dignity as a human being, and to accept his limitations.

The author of the book leaves the wager of the prologue to one side. This is why the 'God' character does not ask Job's forgiveness for having wagered with Satan and allowed him to suffer unjustly. The author is concerned to follow the argument of the body of the book, trying to find a reply to the question of the suffering of the just.

The dialogue between Job and God is mysteriously fruitful. God's earlier silences in the face of the suffering of the innocent made it possible for Job to argue, with wisdom drawn from experience, against the theology that makes the innocent guilty. Although Job did not know it, God was listening to his cries. God's cries, shown by his presence and in his speeches, open Job's understanding: he keeps silent and hears wisdom.

Silences and cries from God can open the way to hope. During God's most penetrating silences, Job almost loses hope: 'Where then is my hope? Who will see my hope?' (17.15); then, in the next speech, he reaches the assurance that his Redeemer lives and that he will see God face to face (19.25–26).

In the epilogue, Job's fortunes are restored. But this restoration is not on account of his not having cursed God despite his adversities. To believe this would mean proving Satan and the comforters right in proposing a God who exchanges restoration for not cursing – upholding the doctrine of retribution.

Job does not curse God, nor does he bless God. He challenges God with the injustice committed against the innocent and the just. God accepts Job's challenge; he neither accuses him nor blames him. Nor does he accept his argument entirely. God is not the one to blame. Simply, like Job, he recognizes the fact. Both recognize their limitations:[5] God's perhaps springs from his infinite mercy even to the wicked (since he does not dare to do away with them altogether, (cf. 40.9–14), and Job's from his littleness and ignorance of this God of grace (40.4; 42.5). Both suffer from this lack of response to the cry of those who complain of violence committed unjustly.

In the text Job's fortunes are restored, but those of the women and men born into the world of destitution, living there and watching Job fall and rise, are not. These are those described in 30.1–10, despised even by Job himself, those who, 'Through want and hard hunger . . . gnaw the dry and desolate ground, they pick mallow and the leaves of bushes, and to warm themselves the roots of broom. They are driven out from society; people shout after them as after a thief. In the gullies of wadis they must live, in holes in the ground and in the rocks. Among the bushes they bray; under the nettles they huddle together. A senseless, disreputable brood, they have been whipped out of the land' (30.3–8). They are those described by the Salvadorean poet Roque Dalton as, 'those always suspicious of everything . . ., the do-anythings, sell-anythings, eat-anythings . . . my compatriots, my brothers'.

The excluded, the target of all 'plagues', are the 'Jobs' of today, whose presence alone, like a crucified body, should terrify humanity. This is why we must not stop crying out demanding justice and why we must know when to keep silent and to experience silences. Thus we shall better discern cries from silences and silences in response to cries.

Job never accepted defeat, in spite of having been the victim of every ill; he mysteriously managed to keep up an unheard of resistance. He did not let his dignity be trampled on. His last cry was uttered upright, emerging from his garbage heap, walking toward God like a prince (31.37).

In the certainty that God listens, we can affirm like Job (even with his heart 'fainting within him'; 19.27): 'I know that my Redeemer lives, and that at the last he will stand upon the earth' (19.25).

Translated by Paul Burns

Notes

1. I look at the text as a literary work, leaving the question of the unity of its composition aside.
2. G. Gutiérrez, *On Job: God-Talk and the Suffering of the Innocent*, Maryknoll, NY 1987, 4.
3. A. Schöckel, *Biblia del peregrino*, 1993.
4. Judicial terminology abounds in the text. Job wants to put God on trial; his friends plead God's case (13.8). See A. Schöckel and J. L. Sicre, *Job*, 1983.
5. Gutiérrez, *On Job* (n. 2), 76.

Leprosy: Untouchables of the Gospel and of Today

Justin S. Ukpong

Introduction

One irony of our contemporary world, which boasts of more scientific and technological advancement than any other age in human history, is that we are still plagued by social ills in a way that negates our technological and scientific gains. For example, while we are able to overcome the physical distance between us and the moon, which was formerly regarded as unreachable, we are still unable to overcome the social distance that society has placed between certain individuals and human groups on the one hand, and the rest of the human community on the other, on the basis of pathological, physical, biological or social conditioning. Thus people suffering from certain diseases and disabilities, and certain categories of people, are excluded from normal social interaction with other people or discriminated against in society, and so are constituted as socially 'untouchable'. The term 'untouchable' has this social connotation throughout this article.

On the basis of pathological conditioning, victims of leprosy and tuberculosis have remained untouchables in spite of current medical advances, as a result of which these diseases can no longer be easily communicated. Because cholera is still a dreaded disease, Nigeria lost its chance of hosting the world youth football championship in 1995 on account of the outbreak of cholera in one small village in the country. Hope of healing is still very far away for victims of AIDS in spite of intense medical research since its identification in the 1980s. Initially, it was associated with homosexuality and intravenous drug abuse, and was popularly concluded to be God's punishment for these offences. But the discovery of heterosexual victims has belied this claim. Initially also, it was thought to have originated from Africa, specifically the central African region, and to have been a disease of monkeys passed on to humans. Today however, things are being seen differently; the theory of its African origin no longer attracts much following, and it is even being questioned whether the HIV virus to which it is commonly attributed is its real cause. Just like AIDS, Ebola and Marburg, two killer diseases with similar viruses, have defied treatment. Since they were first identified in the 1970s, their natural reservoirs and vectors have yet to be discovered. Again like AIDS, they are transmitted in blood – infected blood getting into skin cracks. Unlike the AIDS virus, however, the Marburg virus is also known to be transmitted by *Aedes aegypti* mosquitoes.¹ While medical science is still in search of the facts about the origin and cure of these diseases, they remain highly dreaded and their victims objects of social disgust.

Untouchables regarded as such on the basis of physical, social and biological conditioning are the physically and mentally handicapped, refugees, people discriminated against by reason of caste, ethnic origin, religion and sex. These are 'untouchables' because people do not want to integrate them into their own small 'world' within society.

In the Gospels, we meet different categories of 'untouchables' similar to those in contemporary society – lepers, the blind, the lame, public sinners, toll collectors, Samaritans, oppressed women and so on. These, as is clear from the Gospels, formed the focus of Jesus' ministry. Jesus bent himself over, amidst criticisms, to re-integrate them into society. Today therefore the 'untouchables' in our society pose a serious challenge to Christian witness. It what follows, I intend to explore the ministry of Jesus in relation to the untouchables of his day and point to the challenge it poses to Christian ministry today.

The making of the untouchables of the Gospels

Leprosy, dead bodies whether of human beings or of animals, and bodily discharge were considered very strong sources of pollution by the Jews even up to the time of Jesus, and their victims were expelled from the community. Leprosy was seen as the plague *par excellence* sent by God on sinners. Most often, however, what was regarded as leprosy was some virulent contagious skin disease, not leprosy in the strict sense. In Exodus 9.8–12 leprosy is recorded as the sixth plague that God sent on the Egyptians. In Deuteronomy 28.27, it is one of the curses put on Israel if they refused to obey God and keep his commandments. In Numbers 12.10–15, Miriam is punished with it for criticizing Moses. King Uzziah, though a just ruler, was struck with it till death for not abolishing idolatrous worship in Judah (II Kings 5.4–5). Pollution arising from contact with dead bodies seems to have been considered the worst, since it had to be removed with special lustral water compounded with the ashes of a red heifer (Num. 19.1–20). Bodily discharge included women's menstrual discharge and any blood discharge in women or seminal discharge in men that was an illness (Lev. 15.1–30).

Other sources of pollution included child birth, sexual intercourse, and unclean animals and food items. After childbirth a woman remained unclean for seven days if the child was a boy, and fourteen days if it was a girl (Lev. 12.1–8). Sexual intercourse made both the man and the woman involved unclean till the evening. They became clean again by washing themselves and their clothing (Lev. 15.18). Contact with unclean animals and unclean food items also made a person unclean (Lev. 1.11–47).

Apart from the above cases, there were people who by virtue of their ethnic origin or profession were, in terms of social interaction, placed at a distance by the Jews and so were constituted as 'untouchables' even in the time of Jesus. Such were Gentiles, Samaritans, toll collectors and public sinners. Gentiles were excluded from the Jewish community for associating with things regarded by the Jews as unclean like eating pigs, etc. and for not worshipping the true God of Israel. Samaritans were the inhabitants of the destroyed Northern Israelite kingdom who had intermarried with the Gentiles since the time of the exile. They were therefore not regarded as pure Jews and were treated like Gentiles. Toll collectors whose profession was to collect tolls for the Roman government formed a category of untouchables as a result of the Roman occupation of Palestine. These were well-to-do Jews who purchased from the state the rights to official taxes and dues, and then collected these from the people. They were despised for working for Gentile oppressors of the Jews, for cheating in the process of toll collection, and for frequent association with Gentiles in the normal course of their business. Not only they themselves but also their families were alienated from the rest of the community, and no money from their hands was exchanged.[2] Public sinners like prostitutes and people caught sinning like the woman in John 8.3–11 were treated with scorn and so constituted another class of untouchables.

Except in the cases of sexual intercourse and associating with people and things regarded as unclean, the process of cleansing involved offering an expiatory sacrifice to remove the contamination, and sometimes a sin sacrifice in addition. As particularly the Priestly Writings of the Old Testament reveal, the people of Israel felt bound by a strict religious and ritual connection to its land and the Temple.[3] The result was that any ritual pollution within the community was considered to affect both the land and the Temple also. For this reason, certain sources of pollution were to be removed from the community (Num. 5.2–3), and once a year, a cleansing sacrifice was offered on the Day of Atonement to purify the Temple, the land and the people.

Socio-cultural background

The making of the untouchables of the Gospels is to be understood against the background of the divide between clean and unclean in the Old Testament world-view. Modern social anthropologists see this division as based on the attempt to avoid confusion between what was regarded as normal and what was regarded as an anomaly within a class. It is therefore basically regarded as a matter of social classification that was guarded with rituals.[4]

The clean–unclean divide in the Old Testament had a cultic, not an ethical dimension; it had value in respect of participation in the cult and did not connote the idea of moral guilt except in the sense that in some cases the situation could have been a result of morally sinful action.[5] This must again be understood within the context of a world-view in which the religious and the secular were integrated, and the secular was subordinated to the religious. In such a world-view, participation in the cult became the centre around which individual and national life was organized. So long as the world-view permitted no separation of the secular from the religious, what was a matter of social classification attained a religious and cultic dimension, and exclusion from participation in cult in turn meant exclusion from social interaction. Since association with what was ritually unclean also made one unclean and therefore unfit to participate in the cult, there was a concern to safeguard and maintain the status of being clean. Those who were unclean were therefore rendered socially 'untouchable'.

The untouchables of the Gospels have a few things in common. They were excluded from the Jewish public cult. They were on the fringe of society; they belonged to the underside of history, not to the centre. They were despised, discriminated against and seen as inferior human beings and social misfits. On the other hand, narratives about them in the Gospels portray them as having a singular bravery, courage and faith that took them beyond the boundaries of the social and religious norms of their time. For example, the woman with a haemorrhage threw to the winds all socio-religious caution regarding the ostracization placed on her by her condition and the danger of rendering Jesus untouchable, and made her way through the crowd to touch Jesus (Mark 5.25–34; Matt. 9.20–22; Luke 8.43–48); such was also the courage of the lepers who went to Jesus for healing (Mark

1.40–45; Matt. 8.1–4; Luke 5.12–16; 17.11–19). From their contexts, these narratives do not depict these people as foolhardy or ill-intentioned. Rather, the people are reflected in a very positive light. They are convinced that interacting with Jesus would not only dissolve the boundary that separated them from the rest of the community and make them whole (cf. Mark 5.28), but would not adversely affect Jesus himself.

Jesus and the untouchables of the Gospel

At the time of Jesus the regulations regarding association with the untouchables were very much in force. As a Jew and even more so as a rabbi, Jesus was expected to observe them to avoid being rendered unclean. On the other hand we find that Jesus interacted with and touched lepers (Mark 1.40–45; Matt. 8.1–4; Luke 5.12–16, 17.11–19), that he touched corpses (Mark 5.21–24, 35–43; Matt. 9.18–19, 23–26; Luke 7.11–17; 8.40–42, 49–56), that he did not rebuke the woman who was suffering from a haemorrhage for touching him (Mark 5.25–34; Matt. 9.20–22; Luke 8.43–48), that he admitted toll collectors (Luke 5.27–32) and public sinners (Luke 7.36–50) into his company. What is the christological significance of all this? Certainly in these texts we are face to face with a christology that effects a breaking of the social boundaries that separated the untouchables from the rest of society, a christology that empowers the marginalized in society, and a view of reality that upturns conventional standards of judgment and signals the presence of the messianic age. Let us examine these a little more in detail and see the challenge they pose to contemporary Christian witness.

Breaking of social boundaries

The category of untouchable, whether in the Gospels or in contemporary society, carries with it a social stigma which, like any other stigma, is devastating for the victim's personality. It is a category that revolves around boundaries imposed on people to keep them within specified limits of social interaction. Any violation of the boundaries by those deputed as clean incurs their automatic contamination and exclusion from the rest of the community as well.

As far as we can see from the Gospels, one significance of Jesus' encounters with the untouchables was the breaking of the social boundaries that separated them from the rest of the human community, the consequent removal of the stigma attached to the status, and their reintegration into the society. In every instance of his encounter with the untouchables, Jesus called to radical questioning the conventional attitude towards these people. Some of the stories indicate this very well. For example, the stories of the raising to life of the widow's son at Nain (Luke 7.11–17) and of Jairus' daughter (Luke 8.40–56) show Jesus publicly touching dead bodies, which were regarded as a very strong source of uncleanness. Similarly, in the story of the woman with a haemorrhage (Luke 8.43–48), normal convention would have required a rebuke from Jesus after the woman had publicly confessed her situation. Rather, Jesus confirmed her faith. We find a similar situation when Zacchaeus, a chief tax collector, received Jesus into his house (Luke 19.1–9). Normal convention forbade Jesus to associate with him, but it was Jesus who first signalled the intention to go into Zacchaeus' house. In addition, Jesus' teaching about cleanness and uncleanness, whereby he redefined the idea of ritual uncleanness (Matt. 15.10–20), points to this removal of the boundary between clean and unclean, touchables and untouchables, and the reintegration of all into one human community. In this way Jesus challenged the conventional attitude to the untouchables.

Empowerment of the marginalized

Powerlessness is a characteristic of the untouchables. It is reflected in their look: shabbiness, timidity, helplessness, anxiety, diffidence. This contrasts with the look and air of the powerful – a commanding air, confident bearing, relaxed posture. The untouchables, even if they are in society, do not belong there – they are always reminded of that in one way or another. They do not belong to the centre of history but to the underside of it.

In the narratives of Jesus' encounter with the untouchables things get changed round. Jesus restores the self-worth of the untouchables and thereby positively empowers them for participation in the life of the community. Such encounters are liberating, resulting in a new lease of life for the untouchables. A few examples will illustrate this.

Bartimaeus, the blind beggar at the roadside in Jericho (Mark 10.46–52), on hearing that Jesus was passing by, shouted to Jesus for help, convinced that Jesus could heal him. But because he did not belong in the community, he was scolded and asked to be quiet by the crowd. That he continued shouting until he got Jesus' attention demonstrates his conviction. The moment Jesus took notice of him meant empowerment for Bartimaeus. One who was at the periphery of society now became the centre of attention as Jesus carried on a conversation with him. His self-worth and human dignity were restored; he was healed and reintegrated into the community. The woman who had a haemorrhage is another example (Mark 5.25–34). She went to Jesus with trepidation, yet with faith and courage. She was not supposed to be there, and so she did not openly ask for healing but went secretly. Eventually she became the centre of attention and received a confirmation of her faith instead of a rebuke for defiling Jesus, which she was likely to have feared.

Upturning conventional standards of judgment

In the Gospel narratives involving the untouchables, Jesus is presented as acting in solidarity with them. This was contrary to convention and altogether unexpected. Jesus was not expected to interact with lepers lest he would be rendered unclean; as a rabbi he was not expected to have anything to do with corpses. Bartimaeus was not expected to get the attention of Jesus, hence he was shouted down by the crowd when he called out to Jesus. When a woman was arraigned before Jesus charged with adultery (John 8.2–11), it was not at all expected that he would let her get away with her sin as he did. In all these and other cases, Jesus acted in solidarity with these people and was thereby seen as going against the Law. Yet the same Jesus came to fulfil the Law (Matt. 5.17). Paul gives us an insight to understanding this apparent contradiction.

In the Letter to the Galatians, Paul is at pains to show that the Law had a function to perform in the scheme of salvation history, and this was to lead the people until Christ came (Gal. 3.19). At the coming of Christ, therefore, the function of the Law became fulfilled. It was not meant to, and could not, lead people to Christ, for that is the function of faith (Gal. 3.22–23), neither was it abolished at the coming of Christ.[6] But with Christ a new regime of grace and love that transcends the regime of Law has set in. Jesus' action in respect of the untouchables points to the standard of judging and acting in this new regime.

Jesus, untouchables and the arrival of the messianic age

Jesus' close interaction with the untouchables portended the arrival of the messianic age. In Luke 7.18–23, Jesus presents his 'mighty works' as a testimony to his identity. In the light of the end-time prophecy of Isa. 35.5–6 reflected in the text, Jesus here identifies himself as the eschatological prophet. The text also points to the actualization of the programme of Jesus' ministry which Luke gives in 4.18–23 in the language of Isa. 61.1–2, another end-time prophecy. All these show that with Jesus the messianic age had set in.

The healing of lepers is mentioned in Luke 7.22 in the context of the ills that were to be taken away in the messianic age, even though this disease is not specifically mentioned in the Old Testament prophecies on this subject (cf. Isa. 26.19; 35.5–6; 42.7; 61.1–2). But the inclusion of leprosy here can be plausibly explained by the fact that the promises of the messianic age consisted basically in bringing the good news to the afflicted, among whom would be lepers, the most dreaded of the afflicted. Besides, like most other diseases, leprosy was seen to be directly connected with sin, and therefore to be taken away in the messianic age which had the wiping away of sin as one feature. Thus Jesus' interaction with the untouchables of his time signals specifically the realization of the messianic promise of proclaiming liberty to captives, in this case, those held captive by socially contrived boundaries (Luke 4.18).

Conclusion

Jesus, as we have seen, broke the boundaries that constituted the untouchables of his day, and reintegrated them into the society. By so doing he signalled the arrival of the messianic age. Christian witness today is challenged to bear the marks of this messianic age. It must seek to break the boundaries that society has constructed to constrain fellow human beings in their social interaction. This seems to be the basic challenge that Jesus' interaction with the untouchables of the Gospels presents to us today in the fact of the social stigma attached to people suffering from diseases like AIDS and leprosy, and people who suffer from certain disabilities or belong to certain ethnic groups or caste, that is, people who constitute the untouchables of our day.

Notes

1. See E. H. O. Parry (ed.), *Principles of Medicine in Africa*, Oxford ^{2}1984, 419–22.
2. Cf. O. Michel, '*Telones*', in *Theological Dictionary of the New Testament*, Vol. 8, Grand Rapids 1979, 89.
3. L. Moraldi, *Espiazione Sacrificale e Riti Espiatori Nell' Ambiente Biblico e Nell' Antico Testamento*, Rome 1977, 230–6.
4. Mary Douglas, *Purity and Danger: An Analysis of the Concepts of Pollution and Taboo*, London 1978, 36, 40.
5. Cf. A. Cave, *The Scriptural Doctrine of Sacrifice*, Edinburgh 1977, 97.
6. Cf. H. D. Betz, *Galatians*, Hermeneia, Philadelphia 1983, 107.

The Apocalyptic Beast: The Culture of Violence

Walter Wink

The worldwide network of Powers – nations, corporations, religions, armies, ideologies, institutions, laws and so forth – operates to the disadvantage of the vast majority of people. Keeping people docile and complicit is thus one of the most urgent tasks of the domination system. Those who wish to expose the delusions spun around the public must therefore develop the gift of discernment. For the Powers are never more powerful than when they act from concealment. To drop out of sight and awareness into the general surroundings, to masquerade as the permanent furniture of the universe, to make the highly contingent structures of current oppression appear to be of divine construction, is the genius of their deceptive art. They have armed might at their fingertips, to be sure, but they know, far better than the oppressed, how fragile and potentially impotent it is. Of what use were Philippine army tanks in 1986 when their commanders refused to carry out orders to roll over unarmed civilians? What power was left to the Philippine dictator Marcos when his own pilots refused to bomb non-violent demonstrators and instead defected to a nearby American air base? The mighty prefer, therefore, to rule by means of invisible constraints: unseen filaments tied to the public's arms and legs, and imperceptible spiritual brain-implants causing the masses to will to be what has been made of them.

Delusion (*deludere* – to play with another to his or her detriment) is a confidence game being played on us by the Powers That Be. That game is nowhere more trenchantly exposed than in the surrealistic images of Revelation 12–13.

The delusional apparatus in Revelation 12–13

Of first significance is the fact that the insights in these chapters of the Apocalypse are revelations. John *sees* what for others is invisible (13.1, 2, 11);

what has previously been unseen 'appears' to him (12.1, 3). Discernment does not entail esoteric knowledge, but rather the gift of seeing reality as it really is. Nothing is more rare, or more truly revolutionary, than an accurate description of reality. The struggle for a precise 'naming' of the Powers that assail us is itself an essential part of social struggle.

The seer does not, however, simply read off the spirituality of the empire from its observed behaviour. The situation is more complex. The demonic spirit of the outer structure has already been internalized by the seer, along with everyone else. That is how the empire wins compliance. The seer's gift is not to be immune to invasion by the empire's spirituality, but to be able to discern that internalized spirituality, name it, and externalize it. This drives the demonic out of concealment. What was hidden is now revealed. The seer is enabled to hear his own voice chanting the slogans of the Powers, is shown that these slogans are lies, and is empowered to expel them. He locates the source of the chanting outside, and is set free from it.

What is so striking about the New Testament understanding of the Powers, especially in the light of the esoteric use made of them by later Gnostics, is that it is so exoteric, so lacking in mystifications, secret passwords, occult forces. There are spirits, to be sure, but they are ethereal spirits of real institutions, laid bare by the discerning power of the gospel.

The Roman empire had brought peace to a fratricidal world. It presided over a period of unparalleled prosperity (for the prosperous). Its might was so legendary that a single emissary could prompt surrender. But this façade of magnificence was bought at a horrible price. The revelation that comes to John strips off the mask of benevolence and reveals, beneath it, the true spirit of Rome. It is not at all like beautiful Roma, seated (as the altar of the Gens Augusta in Carthage depicts her) on a pile of surrendered arms with a cornucopia of blessings pouring out on all flesh. He sees, instead, a grotesque and monstrous deformity bent on supplanting God (Rev. 13), or a harlot seated on Rome's seven hills, inviting promiscuous intercourse with the client-kings she has intoxicated with the aphrodisiac of power (17.1–18).

It is a signal achievement to have discerned Rome's monstrous spirit, though certain cynic philosophers may have done as much. What gives John's vision added depth is its awareness that *the domination system transcends its current embodiments.* No regnant Power is even identical with the domination system. There are too many survivals of partnership, too many outbreaks of human decency, too many compassionate, fair-minded people and strong women and equitable laws and humane officials, to achieve pure domination. But behind each regime (symbolized in

Revelation by the beasts from land and sea) stands the ancient system of domination, whose spirit is Satan (symbolized by the dragon).

'And there appeared another sign in heaven: behold, a great fiery red dragon, having seven heads and ten horns and on its heads seven crowns' (Rev. 12.3). This is none other than ancient Tiamat, the seven-headed hydra, the monster of chaos, the mother of the gods in Babylonian mythology. Murdered by Marduk, the god of order, it was from her corpse that the universe was made. This ancient mythological figure was still known to the first century Roman world as Python in Greece, Typhon in Egypt, Lotan in Syria, and as Leviathan in the Old Testament (Job 3.8; 41; Ps. 74.13–14).

There is a fundamental difference in John's vision, however. In Babylonian myth, Tiamat had originally represented chaos, the ultimate threat to the security of the state. What John now sees is that this primordial dragon has come to represent the spiritual principle behind *empire*. Her chaotic functions have coalesced with those of the ruler and orderer, Marduk. Tiamat and Marduk are one. *Now evil is represented, not as the threat of anarchy, but as the system of order that institutionalizes violence as the foundation of international relations.* The new insight here is that order is not the opposite of chaos, but rather the means by which a system of chaos among the nations is maintained. What this vision reveals is that Marduk has not defeated Tiamat after all, for the order won by violent means is a Tiamatic order. The peace gained by violence is anarchic. Violence tends to turn something into the very thing it opposes. Empire is not, then, the bulwark against disorder, but disorder's quintessence.

John the seer also glimpses a figure even older than Tiamat: 'And there appeared a great sign in heaven: a woman clothed with the sun, the moon under her feet, and on her head a crown of twelve stars; she was pregnant, and she cried out from the birth pangs and the torment of bearing her child' (Rev. 12.1–2).

Who is this woman? We may as well abandon all attempts at a narrow definition. She is Mary, the mother of the Messiah (12.5), but she is also Israel, the mother of the messianic hope. From the allusions in 12.14 to the Jerusalem church's flight to Pella during the Jewish War, she is also clearly the Christian church under persecution. Judging from the heavenly symbolism, she also probably evokes Wisdom or the Shekinah (Wisdom 7.29).

But this woman is not simply described in the usual Jewish symbols. She encompasses the history not only of Judaism but of all humanity as well; she is the transfigured Eve, in everlasting enmity with the serpent (Gen.

3.15; Rev. 12.9). And she embodies not only the hopes of Israel but the myths of the pagans. Artemis, too, appears with a crescent moon and stars, Leto wears a veil of stars, and Damkina, the mother of Marduk, is called 'The lady of the heavenly tiara'. So also features of Isis and the constellation Virgo are represented here. Nor do the 'twelve' stars represent just the twelve apostles and twelve tribes of Israel; they are also the twelve constellations in the zodiac. This is an archetypal woman, the Great Mother herself, whose son will end the domination system. She is an image of domination-free existence itself, forced by the dragon to flee 'to the wilderness, where she has a place prepared by God, so that there she can be nourished for one thousand two hundred and sixty days' (Rev. 12.6) – that is, three and a half years, the symbolic half-life of the old order in its countdown to oblivion.

There is nothing ambiguous about this dragon. It represents the spirit of the domination system in its scorched-earth advance through time. This dragon has embodied itself in one empire after another (Dan. 7–8; 11–12), always ready to cast one off for another, always ready to ride the winner, because it is assured that the very means necessary for one empire to defeat another will make the victor every bit as much a child of the Dragon as its predecessor (Rev. 17.15–17). This vision thus puts the lie to the vain belief that the violent overthrow of empire will solve the problem created by empire. Violence can liquidate the current regime, but not this nimble dragon, who leaps upon its exorcists and possesses them each in turn. Thus John warns: 'If you are to be taken captive, into captivity you go; if you kill with the sword, with the sword you must be killed. This is a call for the relentless persistence (*hypomone*) and fidelity of the saints' (Rev. 13.10).

An empire is, by its very nature, a system in a permanent crisis of legitimation. It is not a natural system, but an artificial amalgam held together by force. That is why propaganda is so essential to it. People must be made to believe that they benefit from a system in fact harmful to them, that no other system is feasible, that God has placed the divine *imprimatur* on this system and no other.

The manufacture of idolatry in Revelation 13

In order thus to delude humanity, to achieve a maximal level of stupefaction, the dragon created 'another Beast that rose out of the earth; it had two horns like a lamb, but it spoke like the dragon' (13.11). This is not a natural, earthly, chthonic creature. It is not a deep archetype bursting from the unconscious. It is a wholly artificial creation. It will later be identified as the 'false prophet' (16.13; 19.20; 20.10), whose task it is to persuade people that their salvation lies in the political order. 'It works great miracles . . . and by these miracles . . . it deceives the inhabitants of the earth' (Rev. 13.13–14).

In appearance this second beast is as meek as a lamb – imitating the Lamb who is to rule the nations – but it speaks with the dragon's voice. It is a dragon in sheep's clothing. The second beast is the priestly propaganda machine of empire. 'It exercises all the authority of the first beast on its behalf, and *compels* the earth and its inhabitants to worship the first beast' (13.12). This goes beyond the realm of religious preference and into the domain of religio–political terrorism.

In historical terms, John is alluding to the civic cultus that grew up around the worship of the emperors, which by John's time had become the litmus test to expose the acids eating at the fabric of empire. Anyone suspected of revolutionary designs or subversive thoughts could be required to burn a pinch of incense before the emperor's image, and refusal was punishable by death.

The second beast, therefore, proselytizes by means of a civil religion that declares the state and its leaders divine. This element of power-worship is stressed over and over by John: people 'worshipped the Dragon, for he had given his authority to the Beast, and they worshipped the Beast, saying, "Who is like the Beast, and who can fight against it?"' (13.4); 'it was given authority over every tribe and people and language and nation, and all the inhabitants of the earth will worship it, everyone whose name has not been written from the foundation of the world in the book of life of the Lamb that was slaughtered' (13.7–8); the second beast 'makes the earth and its inhabitants worship the first beast' (13.12); and it can 'cause those who would not worship the image of the [first] beast to be killed' (13.15). Why does the beast demand worship? Why is it not content merely with obedience?

Because the beast knows that the public is fickle; that opinion swings wildly in response to the slightest shifts on the world scene. What is needed is something that can lash loyalty to the mast where it can ride out the waves of social unrest. Ethnic feeling is not enough. Patriotism is not enough. What is needed is worship of the state. That is what nationalism is and has always been. Nationalism is not, in its essence, a political phenomenon; it is a religious one. Only a transcendent cause can induce young men to risk their lives voluntarily in the absence of any conceivable self-interest.

Propaganda is not merely deception, then. It is the manufacture of idolatry. It is not enough that people be misinformed about the nature of the system, for powerful disconfirming truths could easily slip in to shatter such illusions. But *if you can cause people to worship the beast, you have created a public immune to truth.* Worshippers, as studies of cognitive dissonance show, do not surrender their beliefs in the presence of disconfirming facts. They simply adjust their beliefs to neutralize the facts.

We are all too familiar with the trappings of propaganda: the big lie, or the daily small ones; doctored news dispatches and photographs, planted stories, falsified scientific reports, gossip, innuendo, slander. Even more insidious are the misrepresentations of facts carried by the mass media, which avoid stories that contradict the 'elite consensus', even when the data are highly visible, verifiable, and important. Powerful newspapers often simply parrot national policy, even when their reporters are feeding them information sharply at variance with the official picture, as during the Vietnam War.

But propaganda is extremely weak, as is shown by its failure, after forty-four years, to convert people in the Eastern bloc to Communism. Illusion requires incessant repetition in order to mimic the appearance of reality. Propaganda only works through constant reiteration. It is only in quantity that corrupt values, false perceptions and bogus facts can be sold. Truth, on the other hand, though its lot is never easy, makes its way with but a few friends, or even a single utterance. It does not need the apparatus of salesmanship, because reality itself is waiting to confirm it. Hence the power of the beleaguered prophet, or the mothers of the 'disappeared' demonstrating daily in El Salvador, or the witnesses by the tracks where the White Train carried nuclear explosives to Trident submarine bases in the US: normal people with no economic stake never choose to suffer this much *just to lie*.

Breaking free of the delusional system requires, then, not just unmasking the delusions, but a healing of the servile will in the victims. This is the paradox of moral maturity: we are responsible for what we do with what has been done to us. We are answerable for what we make of what has been made of us. Our capitulation to the delusional system may have been involuntary, but in some deep recess of the self we knew it was wrong. We are so fashioned that no Power on earth can finally drum out of us the capacity to recognize truth. However long it must lie buried, or how severely it has been betrayed, truth will out.

When anyone steps out of the system and tells the truth, lives the truth, that person enables *everyone else* to peer behind the curtain too. That person has shown everyone that it *is* possible to live within the truth, despite the repercussions.

The delusory web spun around us can be broken. Everyone is capable of liberation. Most people are not deliberately unjust. Even our current enemies are in some sense victims. Jesus can command us to pray for our enemies, not because it is pious to do so, but because they are potentially capable of recognizing the wrongness of the present system. We must love our enemies because they too have suffered from the Dragon's delusional game.

Vision heals. Mere awareness of the state from which we are fallen is not enough to effect systemic change, but it is its indispensable precondition. Liberation from negative socialization and internalized oppression is a never-completed task in the discernment of spirits. To exercise this discernment, we need eyes that see the invisible. To break the spell of delusion, we need a vision of God's domination-free order, and a way to implement it. For that, we look to God's new charter for reality, as declared by Jesus.

(Excerpted from *Engaging the Powers*, by Walter Wink, Minneapolis: Fortress Press 1992, and used with permission.)

III · The Challenge of the Plague Experience

Plague and its Human Price: Albert Camus, *The Plague*

Norbert Mette

Where people have had to deal with plagues in history, the question what it means to be and act in a human way, and under such extreme conditions, has taken on an unparalleled explosiveness. Is not any kind of humanity automatically done away with when masses of people are delivered over to death and perish? And if those with whom these people come into contact are in all probability threatened by the same fate? And yet there have also been people who, for whatever reason, have risked their own lives so as not to let inhumanity have the last word in such situations.

The kind of spectrum of historical consequences that the epidemics which constantly swept over the population of Europe in the Middle Ages displayed is summed up by the historian N. Bulst, who is regarded as an expert in this sphere, like this:

> Plagues and epidemics provoked hatred and concern on the part of the population in very different ways. In 1321 the lepers in Frankfurt were the victims of mass persecutions because it was alleged that they had poisoned the wells. In turn, in the Middle Ages the Black Death was the occasion for the most violent pogroms in the history of the Jews. The threat of the royal ordinance of 1493 to drown all the syphilitics found in Paris in the Seine is equally significant in this connection. The attempt to escape the plague, interpreted as God's punishment, by public penance, was encouraged by the authorities and largely accepted by the population. The epidemics of pestilence in particular, but also the English Sweat (1529), marked the beginning of such penitential and intercessory processions, which were sometimes maintained for centuries. This coincided with the cult of special saints, who were sometimes new ones (e.g. St Rochus, the helper in time of need). The Christian

commandment to love one's neighbour also led to the foundation of special brotherhoods or orders which made it their particular task to care for particular victims of the plague or to bury those who had died of the plague (e.g. Antonites, Alexians).[1]

The exiling and extermination of those concerned, the search for scapegoats, the flight into religious or occult practices, the organization of love of neighbour – the human forms of behaviour enumerated here can hardly be brought under a common denominator. But in that case what can humanity mean – in a normative sense?

In no other work is this question so much to the fore and is it so intensively grappled with as in Albert Camus's *The Plague*. So we shall discuss the connection between plague and humanity through this 'chronicle', as Camus calls it – as a stimulus to thought and an indication of the problem, but certainly not in terms of possible solutions.[2]

The Plague, which made Camus world-famous in a very short time, appeared in 1947. A first version had already been written in 1943. In 1941, during his stay in Oran in Algeria, Camus had experienced a typhoid epidemic, making observations during it which he worked into this novel. Furthermore, Camus himself suffered from tuberculosis, a renewed heavy attack of which affected him seriously in 1942. But the decisive key to *The Plague* lies in the contemporary political context. In November 1942, Southern France had also been occupied by German troops. Northern Africa, which had been liberated by the Allies, was thus completely cut off from the motherland of France. So Camus, who was in France to recuperate, found it impossible to return to his wife and family. He sought contact with the French resistance movement and then worked with it.

Against this background we can understand how much 'a city afflicted by the plague, which is cut off from the world and whose citizens are put in quarantine, is an appropriate model for the situation in the world as it was at that time: war and occupation, infection by the ideology of the Nazis'.[3] In his novel Camus explicitly makes connections between war and plague – or more precisely, between the reactions of those concerned to both of these, when he writes, 'There have been as many plagues as wars in history; yet always plagues and wars take people equally by surprise . . . When a war breaks out people say, "It's too stupid, it can't last long." But though a war may well be "too stupid", that doesn't prevent it's lasting. Stupidity has a knack of getting its way' (34). But is there no other answer to such stupidity than to accept it as given by fate? Camus declines this question by means of a variety of individuals whom he introduces in his novel, who have completely different attitudes to the plague. There can hardly be a more impressive description of the human price – in many respects – demanded by a plague. Therefore in what follows I shall simply attempt to describe the novel, following it closely and not setting it in the context of Camus' work as a whole and the literary, philosophical and other aspects associated with it.

I. The plague as protagonist

As the title already indicates, the plague is the protagonist in the novel or the chronicle. It is 'the active element, whereas those afflicted by it are only in a position to react'.[4] Camus gives impressive stylistic expression to the powerful difference between the plague and those who are seized by it: 'Camus creates great, impressive images, visions of destruction and downfall of great poetic weight, for the terrifying domination of the plague, its effects and activity. By contrast Camus describes the reaction of human beings – manifold, apparently inappropriately small, which in total can only delay its effect – in a simple, modest striving for preciseness.'[5] Evil is predominantly in control. What can an individual, what can any group of human beings, do against this?

Once the plague had crept into the city through the rats, and more and more people had fallen victim to it, the city was put in quarantine. The chronicler, the fictitious author of this novel, notes: 'Thus the first thing that the plague brought to our town was exile' (60). By so doing it created the optimum conditions to gather 'all its forces to fling them at the town and lay it waste' (117). To achieve this it 'was posting sentries at the gates and turning away ships bound for Oran' (66). How much it finally dominated the city is shown not only by the steadily rising number of dead but also by the fact that it dictated order within the city as a whole, from the lives of individuals to the administration of the whole of public life – i.e. the necessary care for the sick, the disposal of the dead, the taking of precautions, and so on. 'It (viz., the plague) was a skilled organizer, doing its work thoroughly and well' (148). For months it 'never ceased progressing with its characteristically jerky, but unfaltering stride' (211); it 'smouldered in the chests of our townsfolk, fed the fires in the crematorium, and peopled the camps with human jetsam' (ibid.). And even at the end it was the plague, which was gradually 'in retreat all along the line' (219), 'retreating, slinking back to the obscure lair from which it had stealthily emerged' (224) – until the day that would come some time when 'for the bane and the enlightening of men, it roused up its rats again and sent them forth to die in a happy city' (252).

II. Living and dying under the plague

The 'logic of a development' can be made out in the five acts into which Camus divides the dramatic course of the plague. In the course of time this shows the often changing reactions of the population, at any rate as they are recorded by the chronicler, like this:

Initially we have the picture of a fairly homogeneous city: people go about their business and have some enjoyment – in that order. The main thing is to be healthy. Those who do not fulfil this condition, who are sick or die, are left to themselves. Pain, sickness and death are banished from the general perception. According to the chronicler, the citizens had 'not the faintest reason to apprehend' (7) the events which were to unfold in their city. The heralds of the epidemic in the form of rats which perished in large numbers and the first infected and dead people were deliberately suppressed as long as possible. Only hesitantly did the authorities act and take preventive measures.

The closing of the gates of the city which was then ordered by the prefecture is a decisive break. For many people that resulted in a separation from members of their families who were outside the city at the time. That was all the worse since the time of the separation was unforeseeable, and it was difficult even to maintain contact. However, in public people in general tried to keep up appearances and show a lack of anxiety and some cheerfulness.

When the situation continued to deteriorate after a month, the church authorities 'resolved to do battle against the plague with the weapons appropriate to them, and organized a Week of Prayer' (78); the cathedral was regularly full. Then the mood increasingly began to turn to panic. More and more acts of desperation on the part of individuals, e.g. attempts to break out of the city, were a clear indication of this. The heat of the summer further increased the lethargy.

Whereas initially the plague could be limited to the poor quarter of the city, it steadily encroached on the business quarter and the more prosperous quarter of the city too. All were now involved in the great catastrophe. Attempts were made to do what had to be done with the most perfect routine possible: registration of the sick and their segregation, the quarantining of members of the family, and the burial of the dead. Lack of interest and indifference increased with growing exhaustion and disillusionment. Soothsayers and would-be prophets were very much in fashion. 'There was no room in any heart but for a very old, grey hope, that hope which keeps men from letting themselves drift into death and is nothing but a dogged will to live' (213). It took enough strength to keep them up for oneself. Concern for fellow human beings, solidarity, friendship and love went out of the window.

When the plague declined, the people found it extremely difficult to get used to a normal state of existence. Too much had happened, the psychological weariness was too much for it to be possible for joy to return overnight. But finally – at the end of the book – there is an overwhelming festival, the night of redemption.

III. Variations of attitude and behaviour towards the plague

Camus has embodied, to some degree in a model way, quite different forms of attitude and behaviour in the main re-actors of the novel.

First of all mention should be made of the dying, from the caretaker to Tarrou, whose death struggle is portrayed especially intensively. The most impressive scene is certainly the account of the dying child. They all resist as long as they can, rebelling, crying out against the death that is coming upon them. But all medical interventions are to no avail: the pest shows no mercy. For those who are left behind the only question is why innocent people have to die so cruelly.

Conversely there are also those who profit from the plague. Camus embodies these in Cottard. For him as an obtuse outsider, who is evidently to be arrested for black-marketeering and has already attempted to commit suicide, the epidemic brings a welcome and varied reprieve, which at the same time finds an abrupt end with its end. We find a different attitude in Raymond Rambert, the journalist who is staying in Oran to research and who is taken by surprise by the quarantine; he continues to feel himself to be the visiting outsider, who really has nothing to do with the fate of the city; he wants to escape it to his girl-friend, and finally joins the ranks of those who become his friends and fight the plague with every means. And finally mention should be made of Joseph Grand, who at night still pursues his dream of finding fame with a book, and earns his living by day working as a temporary assistant in the city administration. During the plague, every day for two hours he puts the competence this gives him in registering numbers, making card-indexes, calculating and so on, at the disposal of the voluntary sanitary service – an additional task which puts him in a state of constant exhaustion as a result of which he incurs the wrath of his superior. The three main re-actors who stand at the centre of the novel, Pater Paneloux, Jean Tarrou and Dr Bernard Rieux, will be described in more detail.

1. *'Better than his preaching'*: Pater Paneloux

Pater Paneloux was a Jesuit who was highly respected in Oran, even in the circles of these who were indifferent to religion. In a number of public lectures he had proved himself to be a brilliant intellectual who pursued contemporary developments very attentively and who was able to represent himself as 'a stalwart champion of Christian doctrine at its most precise and purest, equally remote from modern laxity and the obscurantism of the past' (78). His real activity was research into Augustine and the African church.

He was asked to give the closing sermon in the framework of the Week of Prayer mentioned above. He retreated to his study for two weeks to prepare this sermon. The narrator depicts it as a rhetorical masterpiece which held the hearers under its spell. The central statement of this sermon is an interpretation of the plague as the scourge of God, with which he metes out to people who have become sinners their due punishment. However, because it comes from God, in the end it brings salvation, since it brings people insight and thus leads them back to God. According to the narrator, this sermon prompted different reactions. Whereas some knelt down and began to change their lives within, others began to fight the plague with all the more determination.

When he was asked, Pater Paneloux finally joined this second group. He joined the voluntary sanitary service. The one who had previously been 'a man of learning' (106) now came into direct contact with victims of the plague. Just as he had wanted to be a leading scholar, now 'he had elected for the place among his fellow-workers that he judged incumbent on him – in the forefront' (180).

The constant experience of death, especially the confrontation with the dying child, also had an effect on his theological thinking. The second of his sermons described in the novel is quite different from the first in tone and content. Certainly the encounter with praxis had shattered his belief in a just divine order. What Paneloux now says that if one wanted to connect suffering with God, consistently one would have to deny him. One can only accept suffering and commend everything to the difficult love of God, an attitude which Paneloux consistently showed on his imminent deathbed, though those around him could not follow him in it.

2. *'A saint without God' – Jean Tarrou*

The voluntary sanitary service which Pater Paneloux joined had been initiated by Jean Tarrou. He had settled in Oran some time previously and evidently could live very well on his private income. When asked what motivated him in the way he spent his time, he indicated that he was concerned to find inner peace. Earlier events in his life had severely shaken his equilibrium. Since then he had been stubbornly striving for holiness and therefore knew that this was never attainable, for everyone was already carrying around the plague in them. In practice the important thing was 'to take the victim's side – to reduce the damage done' (208); in the midst of the sacrifice one could see whether one could gain peace that way.

At the deathbed of this man, with whom a warm friendship had recently bound him, Dr Rieux assessed his life like this: 'Tarrou had lived a life riddled with contradictions, and had never known hope's solace. Did that explain his aspiration towards saintliness, his quest of peace by service in the cause of others?' (237).

3. 'What interests me is being human': Dr Bernard Rieux

Camus depicts the main figure of the novel, Dr Bernard Rieux, as being very like that of Tarrou, and in all the starker contrast to Pater Paneloux. He did not really need to make his own decision to attend to those who were sick of the plague. For it happened simply and easily in the course of doing his professional duties that he was the first to be confronted with the fact of the plague. Certainly at the beginning he did not want to accept this diagnosis which was forced on him by the symptoms of the disease, but then he devoted himself virtually completely to the fight against the plague, to such a degree that in the end he was completely exhausted. That he has to do this is first of all a matter of course for Dr Rieux, since it is part of being a doctor to protect people from death and prevent diseases – in a quite practical way: 'I have no idea what's awaiting me, or what will happen when all this ends. For the moment I know this; there are sick people and they need curing. Later on, perhaps, they'll think things over; and so shall I' (107).

But behind this there is very probably an ethical attitude, though this cannot be described so much in positive as in negative terms: 'When you see the misery it brings, you'd need to be a madman, or a coward, or stone blind, to give in tamely to the plague' (106). To Paneloux's advice to love what one cannot understand Rieux replies passionately: 'And until my dying day I shall refuse to love a scheme of things in which children are put to torture' (178). Even if with this attitude one must reckon with 'a never-ending defeat' (108).

Much as Rieux is concerned with compassion and solidarity and nothing else, in himself too he had discovered how difficult it is to maintain that particularly in extreme situations: 'One grows out of pity when it's useless. And in this feeling that his heart had slowly closed in on itself, the doctor found a solace, his only solace, for the almost unendurable burden of his days. This, he knew, would make his task easier, and therefore he was glad of it' (76f.). One can put up with the plague only when it, too, becomes routine. Nevertheless, this abstraction must not be allowed to gain complete control; one must not lose sight of the specific individual case. For only then – is the doctor's conclusion at the end of his chronicle – can something be learned from the plague despite everything, 'that there are more things to admire in men than to despise' (251).

Nevertheless, despite considerable ideological differences, it is the level of practical commitment that strongly binds the three main re-actors together.

Without wanting to develop this notion further, it might be mentioned in conclusion that for Camus the plague is a metaphor for every possible extreme situation. These extreme situations, however, differ from normal situations only in that they bring out unadorned what is also the case at other times – namely the real concern for humanity in a society. 'But what does that mean – "plague"? Just life, no more than that', remarks the old asthmatic laconically at the end of the book (250).

Translated by John Bowden

Notes

1. N. Bulst, 'Epidemien. II. sozial- und wirtschaftsgeschichtlich', *LMA* III, 2057–60: 2059.
2. Cf. A. Camus, *La Peste*, Paris 1947, here quoted from A. Camus, *The Plague*, Penguin Modern Classics, Harmondsworth 1960; for secondary literature see above all B. Sändig, *Albert Camus. Eine Einführung in Leben und Werk*, Leipzig 1983; id., *Albert Camus*, Reinbek 1995; P. Gaillard, *La Peste – Camus. Analyse critique*, Paris 1972.
3. H. Lottmann, *Camus, eine Biographie*, Hamburg 1986, 220.
4. Sändig, *Camus* (n. 2), 105.
5. Ibid.

The Christian Ethic: Help or Hindrance?
The Ethical Aspect of AIDS

Marciano Vidal

1. General overview

Within the broad meaning attached in this issue of *Concilium* to the word 'plague, I am tackling a specific issue in the present situation: the AIDS pandemic and the way this disease represents, in current general thinking, the most typical expression of what we understand by 'plague' today. In fact, the slogan 'return of the plague' has come out of society's experience of the disease known as AIDS.

We had thought the plague cycle had come to an end in human history. This belief has evaporated over the last decades; for the last sixteen years (since 1981) we have been faced with a new pandemic that, despite the huge resources deployed, is still resistant to any effective therapy. AIDS is a pandemic – the 'ultimate epidemic' – still looking for a corresponding vaccine.

In using the term AIDS I am referring to the whole process of which the significance and experience of the disease is made up: the existence of the virus (HIV), which can be detected by a test for antibodies; the transmission of this virus to other human organisms, infecting them by three principal methods – seminal and vaginal fluids, blood, the mother-child relationship during pregnancy; the course of the virus in infected persons (HIV-positive); and the final onset of the disease through the 'syndrome' of various nosological processes brought on by 'acquired immune deficiency'.

The reality of AIDS has many aspects. I am not only alluding to the 'many faces' of those infected underlying the term. I am also – and here mainly – referring to the effects this pandemic is having on the global human situation. The following aspects can be distinguished:

– *Economic and financial*: in connection with AIDS (research, manufacture of condoms, publicity campaigns, production and sale of medicines, hospital admissions, health insurance) vast sums are spent, huge businesses – and even organized mafias – have grown up. In Brazil, there is a legal battle going on to force private health insurance policies (virtually obligatory since there is no national health insurance) not to exclude AIDS from their cover: the insurance companies do not want to take on the burden because it is costly and not profitable.

Blood and plasma banks have also become a huge international business (remember the contaminated plasma in France) and in some countries such as Brazil transfusions have been a major cause of the spread of AIDS. There, a great national campaign was mounted to make blood banks more strictly accountable under the law, but as financial resources are scarce, the contamination continues.

– *Social*: I summarize three points that appear more fully in some form in the main body of this article. 1. The prevalence of ignorance and illiteracy leads to many people becoming infected, normally through cheap prostitution. The AIDS epidemic is spreading fast among young, poor and ignorant women who take to prostitution as a means of survival. They are obviously equally transmitting agents, since their ignorance and the *machismo* of their clients, who refuse to use condoms, create the conditions for the spread of the disease. 2. There is great growth in the number of HIV-positive children who lose their already infected mothers: these are the orphans of AIDS, and the church is virtually the only agency taking on their care. 3. Many are being dismissed from their jobs because they have AIDS.

– *Media*: The communications media, TV in particular, carry most of the publicity campaigns designed to combat the disease – often lacking in human and ethical content. The media also transmit prejudices and a culture of discrimination against the victims, but have also been responsible for campaigns of solidarity and enlightenment.

– *Scientific*: There is a need to continue analysing the structure and mutations of the HIV virus and its source, as well as classifying the derivations that arise in the final phase of AIDS.

– *Technological*: The main objective is to discover an effective vaccine; in the meantime, the need is to provide the most effective and humane palliative and life-prolonging therapies.

– *Political*: As a disease with huge social implications, AIDS demands special attention on the part of world and national authorities to provide the necessary resources, objective information, educational and public health programmes, and the corresponding legislation.

– *Professional*: Health professions are challenged by AIDS not only in their curing, but also in their caring function.

To these basic aspects there have to be added others no less important from the human standpoint: the *personal* aspect, the *family*, the *charitable*, the *pastoral*. AIDS not only has many 'faces' and many 'aspects' but is also a 'challenge' to all: individuals, families, professionals, scientists, administrators, society, churches.

Can one also speak of an *ethical* aspect? Evidently one can, but not every type of moral consideration is appropriate. Hence the title of this article, alluding to the double and contradictory role ethics can play: *help* or *hindrance*. What follows is an assessment of the basic conditions for a correct ethical, and specifically Christian ethical, approach to the question of AIDS.

2. Ethics as 'help' and not 'hindrance'

The first condition for ethics, both in practice and in discourse, to be a help and not a hindrance in overcoming AIDS, is for it to be freed of all ideological manipulation or instrumentalization. The history of morality provides many forms and situations of instrumentalization of ethics aimed at inducing specific behaviour by utilizing the mechanisms of fear, anguish and threat of punishment in this life and/or the next. Resorting to this kind of threat has not been absent from moral discourse on AIDS.

The presence of AIDS has been attributed to moral relativism, to present-day permissiveness, especially sexual permissiveness, and to lack of religious faith. This unwarranted connection between AIDS and immorality has sought to uphold postures of assigning 'moral responsibility' to the victims and rejecting the just moral autonomy achieved over the past decades.

The ethical dimension is also manipulated when it is formulated in tabooistic heteronomous terms. It is a tabooistic understanding of ethics to hypostasize 'nature' and think the AIDS disease nothing other than the 'vengeance' of a wounded and violated natural order. Heteronomous understandings are those that project a 'victimist' and 'propitiatory' ethic on those suffering from the disease: thinking that they have to bear the punishments indissolubly linked to transgression of the moral order.

To free itself from ideologizing instrumentalization ethics has to set itself on the only foundation that gives rise to objectivity and impartiality – the truth. It is ignorance, above all 'affected' ignorance, that generates unfounded fears, susceptible to manipulation. The truth about AIDS, which has to be the foundation for moral discourse on it, is concentrated on three main areas:

1. *What it is*. It is, basically, a disease, and has to be treated as such. All other considerations, concerning its cause or concerned to make value judgments, are exposed to unwarranted falsifications and extrapolations.

2. *How it is transmitted*. In the face of alarmist ideas on the means and methods of infection, we need objective information. We know that transmission routes of AIDS can be reduced, as I noted above, to three main ones: sexual intercourse, blood contact, mother–child relationship.

3. *How to prevent it*. Prevention has to be located in behaviour linked to the three main routes of infection. Indiscriminate and promiscuous sexual practice, both homosexual and heterosexual, provides a propitious setting for the transmission of HIV, especially when precautions are not taken. The same applies in situations linked with blood contact: professional practice, particularly medical; blood transfusions; and, above all, sharing syringes among drug addicts. Pregnancy in HIV-positive women carries a high risk of transmitting the virus to the child.

The ethical dimension of AIDS is not something heteronomous to its reality, condemnatory and threatening in tone. On the contrary, it is based on that same reality and tries to convert 'truth' into 'moral commitment'. Modes of behaviour will be moral in so far as they stem from truth and seek to embody truth. The three areas of truth about AIDS, just listed, constitute so many essential reference-points for the ethical dimension.

Another condition for ethics being a 'help' and not a 'hindrance' is that the moral dimension must be connected with the other aspects of AIDS. One cannot speak of ethics as a separate entity: moral discourse must always be a discourse referred to the other dimensions of the question. Ethics operates as an axiological dimension, bringing responsibility to bear on the scientific, technological, political, professional, charitable and personal aspects of AIDS. As such, it does not remove autonomy from these other dimensions but, on the contrary, supports the particular function each of them has, while guiding all of them toward the general and convergent objective of the greatest and best human good (individual and collective), an integrating viewpoint that corresponds to proper moral consideration.

3. Basic criteria of the ethics of AIDS

If I had to synthesize the ethical aspects of AIDS, I should not hesitate to arrange them around two basic criteria. The first aims principally at the subjective dimension of morality: this is the criterion of 'responsibilization'. The second has to do with the objective aspect: this is the criterion of 'non-discrimination'.

(i) The criterion of 'responsibilization'

The basic standpoint of the ethics of AIDS is that of responsibility. For practical purposes, moral discourse is identical to analysis of human responsibility in the three decisive stages of AIDS: that of prevention, that of transmission, and that of healing (care and resources). There are many responsible subjects implicated in these three stages: scientists, health professionals, government, sufferers, the whole of society. To a particular degree, responsibility is concentrated on behaviour associated with the transmission of HIV; importance also attaches, however, with regard to 'responsibilization', to the actions of professionals, politicians and the whole of society in its dealings with sufferers and the search for a means of eradicating the disease.

So, then, the prime function of ethics in this regard is to raise the level of responsibility in everyone connected with AIDS. This responsibility presupposes precise understanding of the disease (what it consists of, how it is contracted, and so on), but it also requires the effective implication of the freedom of the individual. AIDS will be eradicated, or at least will become more bearable, only when the degree of human responsibility involved in it is raised. In fact, the best method of preventing AIDS is responsible and well-informed behaviour.

(ii) The criterion of 'non-discrimination'

Besides making people more responsible, ethics has the aim of putting forward a project of humanization in the dehumanized and dehumanizing situation of AIDS. As in all ethical discourse and all moral practice, what is being pursued in the ethics of AIDS is the recovery and raising of the integral well-being of those implicated.

In order to achieve this objective of humanization, ethics sets out an agenda with two decisive stages. In the first place, it provides an overall view to make the phenomenon of AIDS understandable. This overall view is made up, in the first instance, of the data provided by distinct areas of knowledge of the disease in question; but it also contains the axiological reference-points of the individual: an end in him/herself, an absolute value. Furthermore, the religious – and specifically the Christian – standpoint helps to fill in the overall meaning by situating the disease and its sufferers under the gaze of the good God and under the influence of the suffering and risen Christ.

It is then necessary to deduce the estimations, attitudes and behaviour corresponding to this overall view. This whole complex of estimative preferences, attitudes and specific behaviour is, in the case of AIDS, organized around a criterion that, in negative form, can be expressed as 'non-discrimination'. In positive terms, it is the criterion of inclusion in solidarity. For human responsibility in the face of AIDS to acquire a valid objective, its starting point and desired goal has to be the criterion of acceptance of the 'other' (in this case, the possible or actual sufferer from AIDS) as a someone whom I cannot 'shut out' but must, on the contrary, 'bring in' in a special way to the dynamic of solidarity of human actions.

The double criterion of responsibility and non-discrimination is verified in the specific areas comprised in the overall situation of AIDS. These areas form so many headings within the practical morality of AIDS. An 'ethical *summa*' of AIDS has to take the following headings into account:

– *Social ethic*: critique of the mentalities, attitudes, and behaviour currently prevalent in society; proposal for an alternative based on truth and non-discrimination.

– *Political-governmental ethic*: allocation, on a just and proportionate level, of resources for research; respect for truth and for personal and social well-being in information, education and public health policies; proposal for adequate and just legal measures.

– *Professional ethic*: moral obligation to care for the sick; responsible actions in professional practice (testing for antibodies, monitoring the course of the disease); secrecy and confidentiality combined with giving the due amount of information to the sick; non-discriminatory attention and care.

– *Personal ethic*: appeal for responsibility in behavioural patterns related to transmission of or infection with the disease, applied to oneself and to other people.

Rather than expound this whole complex of ethical requirements in different ways under each specific area, I prefer to allude to the specific implications of the two basic criteria I have set out. The criterion of non-discrimination refers more to the care of the sick and preventing the propagation of the pandemic. That of 'responsibilization' is more orientated prevention of infection. These are the two ethical messages I wish to comment on in the following sections.

4. The ethical message of non-discrimination

The spontaneous reaction to any epidemic has been, and still is, a tendency to establish mental and physical mechanisms of 'exclusion' or 'discrimination', operating against the sick. Faced with this primary attitude, we have to provoke a human decision to 'include' the disease and its sufferers in the normal channels of acceptance in togetherness. One of the essential messages of an ethics of AIDS is, as I have said, that of non-discrimination. Let me now list the commonest situations in which mechanisms of 'exclusion' operate and which, as a result, require a moral effort to solidarity and inclusion.

(i) In social concepts

AIDS is a fact that, like all broadly and deeply significant acts in human life, gives rise to social concepts. AIDS is a great metaphor in which social mentalities are condensed and which gives rise to induced social behavioural patterns. To a large extent, AIDS has now become the symbolic place into which social concepts of discrimination all flow together. It is also the opportunity for building the symbolic human space for inclusion in solidarity.

The following social mentalities and attitudes belong to the pole of discrimination:

– *Stigmatizing particular social groups*. The expression 'groups at risk' carries this discriminatory charge. With it, we 'mark out' (exclude) mini-collectivities, such as homosexuals and drug-addicts, seeking to exclude them (expel them) from the body of society.

– *Hiding or privatizing the disease and the sick*. As it is considered something 'shameful', every effort is made to hide the disease. The mental mechanism of privatization is often used to this end: 'It's his problem' (the sick person's), 'It's nothing to do with me'. It is not difficult to glimpse a presumed superiority on the part of the non-infected person in this attitude, and even a hidden pleasure in the harm suffered by the 'other'.

– *Demonizing the sick*. For an excluding social mentality, the sick are real or potential enemies. They become agents through which evil is diffused in society; they are, therefore, a demonic force that disturbs social cohesion.

– *Projecting a generalized guilt on to the disease and those suffering from it*. The disease and the sick are enveloped in a 'victimist' and 'expiatory' mentality. The sick are victims of their sins; the sickness is their expiation of their sinful behaviour.

This concept of discrimination and exclusion normally gives rise to the same sort of actions in society. These include: rejection of HIV-positive children by schools; having to hide the presence of people with AIDS in residential districts for fear of the adverse reaction of neighbours; exaggerated precautions, taken out of unjustified fear of infection, in particular workplaces or services, such as hairdressers, barbers, and the like.

In the face of this social concept of exclusion and discrimination we have to propose a social ethos of acceptance and inclusion – and put it into effect. The first thing that has to be asked of an ethics of AIDS is that it stress the basic moral principle of humanity: to treat 'the other' as an 'I', that is, to include everyone in the 'realm of ends in themselves' (Kant), in which a same absolute value obtains for every human being.

These statements are clearly underscored by the ethical discourses not only of Kant but of present-day philosophers such as Paul Ricoeur and Emmanuel Lévinas. Their deeper foundation is the root human moral sensitivity expressed through the rule of ethical reciprocity (the so-called 'Golden Rule'): treat others as you would wish them to treat you, 'Do as you would be done by'. Furthermore, the Christian world-view supports, guides and gives substance to this ethical alternative of inclusive solidarity by insisting that those suffering from AIDS are children of God and members of the mystical body whose head is Christ.

(ii) In political public health measures

Those suffering from AIDS, like any human group 'marked out' by the stigmas of marginalization or dangerous 'difference', run the risk of seeing their rights as citizens diminished. I refer specifically to particular political decisions in the field of public health as well as to actions on the part of medical professionals.

It is clear that various governing bodies, national and international, have the duty to safeguard the common good on the national and international levels. Specifically, they have to devise and carry out effective programmes aimed at controlling, reducing, and – within the measure of the possible – eradicating the spread of the AIDS disease. This objective requires legal, public health, educational, and publicity measures, as well as support for research.

Ethics is not only not opposed to but actively supports such interventions as tend to promote and safeguard the common good. Nevertheless, we must not fail to denounce the potentially (and in some cases actually) discriminatory measures that form part of political and administrative decisions and of certain actions carried out by health professionals. To list some such measures:

Indiscriminate obligation to take an antibodies test: on immigrants, prostitutes, drug-addicts; as a general measure on incoming prisoners; as a condition for receiving a bursary for study (exercised above all on students of African origin); as a requirement for certain posts in public service.

Not guaranteeing those HIV-positive and suffering from AIDS the basic rights of every citizen: to work, to state as well as private insurance, to freedom of travel and residency.

Cutting down their entitlement to health care.

Discriminatory isolation of AIDS-sufferers in hospitals and clinics: the disease is not infectious through mere proximity, and so isolation is not necessary; it only makes sense if it is in the interest of the AIDS-sufferers themselves.

5. The ethical appeal to responsibility

Next to the ethical value of non-discrimination, we have to situate the appeal to responsibility. These two moral references – non-discrimination and responsibility – form the two primary objectives of an ethics of AIDS.

Responsibility is a requirement of all human behaviour. But it is more so in actions related to epidemics. The history of these shows that humankind has conquered disease not only through vaccines but also through heightened responsibility. The interaction between the advance of technical medical knowledge and human responsibility in behaviour has been the most effective means of overcoming plagues throughout history.

The appeal to responsibility becomes even more necessary in the case of AIDS, since this disease belongs to the category of 'moral diseases' as classically defined by Hippocrates. 'Moral' here does not have its strong sense but that which derives from *mores* (customs, behaviour). That is, it is not a disease whose cause is merely 'natural' but one occasioned by particular 'customs' or behavioural patterns.

Responsibility has to enter into all the agents, factors and situations intervening in or making up the human phenomenon of AIDS. Specifically, there has to be:

Responsibility in research: this must be carried out not merely for scientific or economic ends, nor by utilizing the mechanisms of an exaggerated competitiveness, but with the good of people as its primary objective;

Responsibility in publicity, educational, legal and preventive policies: these must not overstep the bounds of objective truth, even with the good intention of making the populace more aware, nor must they violate the rights of individuals through seeking short-term results or taking shortcuts;

Responsibility in professional practice: possible errors in diagnosis (through a test for antibodies) must be eliminated, and all the possibilities of cure or palliation must be pursued; errors in transfusions of blood plasma infected with HIV are most regrettable.

While these areas of responsibility are most important, I believe that responsibility associated with personal behaviour is even more so. The appeal to responsibility on the part of those directly implicated in AIDS has to lead these people to behave in a well-informed and deliberate manner in the three situations that can produce infection and in which, therefore, preventative measures have to be taken:

Responsibility in sexual behaviour: they should know that a controlled sex life is the most effective measure;

Responsibility in drug-addiction: they should realize that sharing needles is a virtually certain route to infection;

Responsibility in procreation: they should accept that the right to procreate has to be limited by the obligation not to transmit such a transcendental disease as AIDS to their children.

This is not the place to embark on a detailed discussion of ways and means of exercising responsibility in these three areas. I would only remark that ethics has to distinguish between the ideal and the actual possibilities in situations which, in most cases, involve people 'deteriorated' through drug-addiction, social marginalization (prostitution), or the anomalies of sex life.

Bearing in mind the tension between the ideal and actual possibilities, the need to prevent infection among drug-addicts should be resolved pragmatically, sometimes by giving them clean syringes; there is nothing to be gained, in my view, by the hypocrisy of some penitential establishments, which, because they do not 'officially' recognize that drugs are available in them, do not supply any effective means of preventing the supply of the epidemic.

In cases where HIV-positive women are liable to become pregnant, they should be offered every means, short of abortion, to prevent a procreation that would be totally irresponsible.

Catholic ethics has questioned the use of condoms to prevent infection with HIV. Some theologians have taken the view that the use of condoms is to be indiscriminately condemned in all cases. It seems to me that we should distinguish some situations from others. In the case of behaviour contrary to official Catholic morality (heterosexual sex outside marriage, homosexual sex) it is preferable not to add a 'greater evil' (infection) to an already immoral act if it can be prevented through the use of a condom. And when behaviour is 'correct', as in the case of intercourse between married partners one of whom is HIV-positive, it does not seem incorrect to use condoms as a 'lesser evil' in order to prevent greater ones.

Translated by Paul Burns

Seeds of Hope

Zilda Arns Neumann

Introduction

The progress made in theological interpretations and scientific discoveries helps us to understand that the presence of plagues in the modern world should not be seen as punishment for sins committed. They should rather be viewed in the context of our common responsibility for social structure, where we need to play an active part in the work of human formation aimed at developing our affective, spiritual, intellectual, and physical potentialities and building up an equality of opportunities that leads to social justice and peace.

Children do not look to an improvement in the conditions of life and education of the families into which they are born as a springboard for their development, but child-care, particularly in adverse situations, is a major determining factor in future changes to the quality of life of the whole of society. The period in a child's life from gestation to the age of six is the most important phase of its life, when its way of behaving, of relating, of developing its human values and potential, are all being worked out. When society becomes involved in child-care for this age-group, it discovers that the context of child-care work is more all-embracing, because children depend on the well-being of their families, which suffer the consequences of the execution of public policies, which in turn depend on social organization. In this context, plagues are the result of living and organizing society in a way that does not collaborate in improving the quailty of life of all. So it generates violence, mainly because children maltreated when small carry a germ of violence within them for their whole lives.[1]

In the Old Testament we meet a person who had the ability to read the signs of the times; his name was Moses. He saw the unjust system and the social inequality bearing on the Hebrew people in a situation of slavery. Before the liberation of the people of Israel, all were afflicted by a series of plagues, including the death of first-born sons, which threatened the very continuance of life. History is repeating itself, with the difference that today every Christian community is better equipped with the knowledge that can enable it to understand and combat most of our plagues.

1. My personal experience of combatting plagues

Here I should like to describe the best experience of my life as a Christian and a professional health worker. At the outset of my professional career, or rather while I was still adolescent, I chose medicine; as a catechist at the time, I was also extremely concerned over what seemed an unbridgeable dualism: my actions in the world as a doctor, and what I did as a Christian. I dreamed of travelling the long rivers of Amazonia by boat and of leaping the hillocks and pits of the slums of the big cities, curing the sick; I felt within me a strong sense of vocation, of personal and professional achievement, of the grace of God, who can do all things. At the same time, God's ways to this personal achievement proved very different: a widow with five children, with more than twenty years of professional experience in administering programmes of mother-and-child health care, I came up against another side of life. I came into contact with widows who had no work and no house, women abandoned with no idea how to remedy their sad situation. I knew too from experience that good health-care projects could be overturned, with no redress, simply to punish a good administrator who had taken part in some demonstration by an opposition party. It was at this crossroads in my life, in September 1984, that God called me, through the offices of my brother, Cardinal Paulo Evaristo Arns of São Paulo, and with my companion on this journey, the then archbishop of Londrina, Geraldo M. Agnelo, who was then a member of the Episcopal Pastoral Council of the National Conference of Brazilian Bishops (CNBB), to put into effect a dream, which became a reality, the Pastoral Child-care Office of the CNBB. As a Christian, I felt called by Jesus Christ to be salt of the earth and light of the world, and God would complete the work.

As a paediatrician and sanitarian, I was convinced that plagues such as diarrhoea, pneumonia and other respiratory infections, low birth-weight, premature births, malnutrition, and even poverty and domestic violence, could be minimized if there were someone to support mothers, giving help when it was most needed. My more than two dozen years' professional experience in care of children, adolescents and mothers, administering governmental and non-governmental agencies for mother-and-child help, health centres, mothers' clubs, and other bodies, had left me with a strong feeling of the need for 'angels' to stand alongside families and help them in preventing diseases, stresses, violence – usually easily avoidable.

One thing always worried me: in government, people could do many things, devise many programmes, but it was always difficult to reach the poorest communities; public services found it hard to go out to meet families, to enter into the intimacy of their decision-making processes. They were organized in ways designed to attract the broad population, but the poorest families lacked the 'steam', the energy, to follow such programmes; they were left by the wayside. My Christian side began to show me solutions. In the distance, I discerned solidarity, Christian mysticism, giving strength to the church's social commitment; in practice, the unity between faith and life could help to save thousands and thousands of lives if the gift of knowledge were shared among neighbours in deprived communities.

It was clear to me that poverty, poor living conditions, poor education, poor public health, were the main cause of these avoidable deaths. Besides combatting poverty, it was absolutely necessary to care for people's education and health; this meant going to community leaders and, among them, especially to women in their family context, to teach them to manage the basic processes of health care, nutrition, and development of their children; to raise their self-esteem and that of their children. Developing Christian fraternity and solidarity among people in a practical and organized manner, in order to combat infant mortality, malnutrition and domestic violence, would be the vital instrument for success. To guarantee enthusiasm and perseverance in this voluntary work, three areas were in need of constant encouragement: the development of pastoral leaders, giving them ever-increasing resources for their mission; strengthening people's sense of belonging to one united family; making Jesus Christ visible as the reference-point for their life and work. This last was perhaps the deepest secret of the increase in new leaders each year, with thousands engaging in this struggle in the service of life and health.

My professional experience, aided by my background in a large family, enabled me to map out the routes to be followed along the way: democratization of knowledge, simplified techniques for popular understanding and mastery. This methodology was inspired by the Gospel 'sharing of loaves and fishes', as recounted by the apostle John. After being lifted up to heaven, for small organized groups, science can also be shared out in the same way and, with a final appraisal of the results of this endeavour, there will still be baskets full of knowledge and good will to be gathered up. Empowering community leaders, so that they would share all they knew with their neighbours, becoming a resource for mothers and families, would be the dorsal fin of this undertaking.

The Good Shepherd's example taught us to prioritize high-risk children and families – the hungry, the unemployed, prostitutes, drug addicts, slum-dwellers in the *favelas* round the big cities, in rural areas, and in indigenous zones. To help everything run as smoothly as possible, St Paul taught us that every person should be stimulated to use the gifts he or she had, and then not to work alone, because if one became discouraged, another would step in with encouragement. So it was important to work in groups and communities, so that no individual or family would feel alone, thereby creating the habit of seeking help from other people, from the neighbourhood, the community.

2. Seeds of hope

That is how 'Pastoral Child-care' came into being in 1983. And this is what happens: instructed volunteer community leaders weigh all children under the age of six living near them; others teach alternative cooking methods to improve nutritional standards through making good use of regional products; others teach the use of home-made serum to combat the dehydration caused by diarrhoea, practise the use of medicinal herbs to combat respiratory diseases, look after pregnant women so that children will be born healthy and loved; they encourage breast-feeding, the first school of love, companionship and dialogue; they teach and weigh the children, making the 'weighing day' a day of celebration of 'the life of the community', and promoting the basic skills needed to ensure that infants develop properly. Vaccines, which have cost millions of dollars in research and are still not appreciated by many families, are another priority concern. Some leaders learn how to listen to complaints and to make people live at peace with themselves and with others. Others use their natural gifts to teach people who to earn enough to enable their families to survive; still others teach reading skills to children and adults. An outstanding contribution is made by the 'From Womb to Six' programme of catechesis, which sets out a way of uniting faith and life in a context of love. The development of social communications to encourage people along the way, promoting an exchange of skills and experiences and influencing the conduct of basic public policies dealing with social management and everything necessary for the promotion of life, has been an area on which we have concentrated most in recent years.[2]

(i) The social context

The peripheries of the big cities and the pockets of deprivation in the small and medium municipalities, in towns and in the countryside, are the scenario for the activities of Pastoral Child-care. Today, more than 111 million Brazilians are crowded into the big cities, as a result of the occupation and exploitation of rural land. As a result, there is extreme

The Reach of Pastoral Child-Care

Fourth quarter 1996 (1)

States (100%)	27
Municipalities with Pastoral Child-care (49%)	2,519
Regions of the CNBB (100%)	16
(Arch)dioceses or Prelacies (98%)	248
Parishes registered (42%)	3,874
Communities registered	21,595
Acting community leaders	78,937
Families accompanied (2)	2,049,272
Pregnant women accompanied (2)	137,506
Children under six accompanied (2)	3,025,077
Alternative Community Projects for income generation (3)	1,178
Radios with 'Long live Life' programmes	853
Literacy Groups for young people and adults (4)	1,114
Students enrolled in literacy courses	17,867

(1) Preliminary data for communities whose 'Accompaniment records' had reached the National Coordination Centre by 19 Feb. 1997
(2) The numbers of families, children and pregnant women refer to the fourth quarter of 1996.
(3) Mutual Aid, Income Generation, and Occasional Assistance projects approved by 27 Feb. 1997.
(4) Literacy projects for young people and adults approved by 27 Feb. 1997.

poverty and deprivation on the peripheries of these cities, while the situation of families who cling to the rural areas is not very different.

An account prepared by Itamaraty and presented to the meeting of the World Forum for Social Advancement held in Denmark in 1995 listed 42 million people living in poverty in the country, of whom 16 million live in utter destitution. The figures show that around 6.3 million poor Brazilians are children under the age of five, and that 2.4 million of these live in conditions of absolute deprivation. These children are the main victims of family breakdown, mostly caused by unemployment, lack of housing and security, constant migration, and also absence of or difficulty of access to basic health and education services. On top of this age-group are the other children, the adolescents and the women, equally victims of this situation of extreme poverty.

This is why the activities of Pastoral Child-care are aimed principally at families in need, which suffer from the major problems deriving from lack of access to social and cultural benefits, and in which infant mortality is highest, accounting for 229,000 deaths at under five every year (UNICEF-SMI, 1997).

Present throughout Brazil, the Pastoral Child-care arm of the CNBB's Social Action organization is recognized as one of the most important organizations in civil society, certainly the largest in the world working in health, nutrition, and education of children from gestation to six years of age, deliberately involving families and communities. Around 5,000 support and co-ordination teams, made up of volunteers, work alongside the community leaders.

(ii) A flexible structure

The structure of Pastoral Child-care – National Coordination Centre; State, Diocesan, Parochial, and Community Coordination Centres – is as simple and flexible as possible. Around seventy per cent of the resources provided by the National Coordination Centre, besides special instruction courses and educational materials – videos, strip cartoons, primers designed and tested at national level – are administered directly by the dioceses, which pass them on to parishes and communities where they can be directed to the families in need.

Diocesan Coordinators render accounts to the National Coordination Centre, which concentrates the administration and decentralizes all activities and resources, with computerized records giving immediate access to the financial and material resources needed for each project. This efficiency in the central management of Pastoral Child-care is one of the guarantees of the success of its activities in a country the size of Brazil.

(iii) Results

Small miracles are being accomplished on a daily basis. Whereas Brazilian government agencies (IPBG/IPEA) are projecting that by the year 2000 infant mortality through the country will have fallen to 39.2 per

Mortality Reduction among Children under the Age of One accompanied by Pastoral Child-care

Brazil and the North-East, 1992–1996

Mortality rate for those 'accompanied' compared to previous year

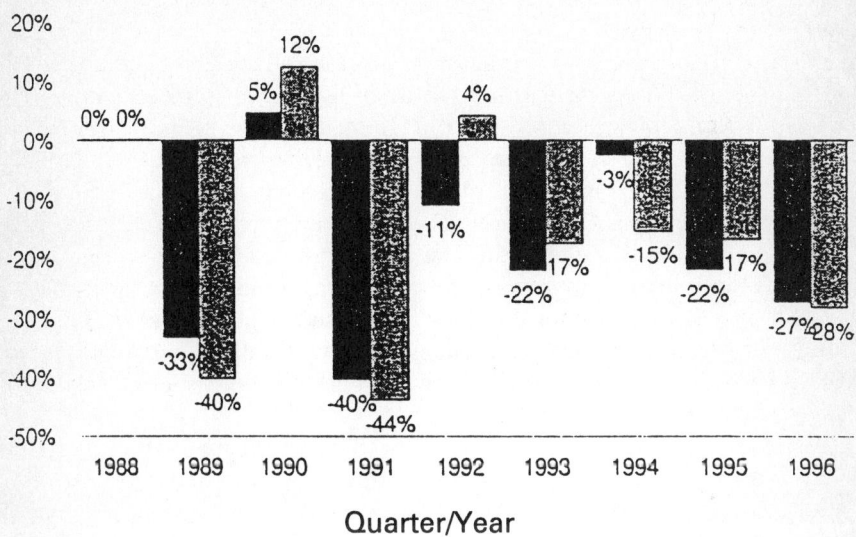

% Reduction
■ Brazil
☒ North-East

SOURCE: Pastoral Child-care/CNBB, Accompaniment Records and Monthly Appraisals of the Basic Activities of Health, Nutrition, and Education in the Community, delivered to the National Coordination Centre in Curutiba, up to 19 February 1997.

1,000 live births, Pastoral Child-care has already reduced the number of infant mortalities to between 18 and 28 per 1,000 in the deprived communities where it is present. These results are all the more significant when one remembers that it acts exclusively in the pockets of greatest poverty and deprivation, in which the rate of infant mortality is usually more than double the national average.

Within the activities of the national programme for the reduction of infant mortality coordinated by the Brazilian government in cooperation with non-governmental agencies, Pastoral Child-care has intensified its activities in the 217 municipalities, spread over 20 states, which IBGE/UNICEF have identified as high-risk for infants. In just two years of activity, this action resulted in a drop in infant mortalities from 100.5 to 35 per 1,000 live births. This result was possible thanks to the effective actions of 6,447 Pastoral Child-care agents 'accompanying' 245,489 infants in these municipalities.

Other results deserving of mention are the reductions in violence and marginalization, and the return of 'attended' families to ethical values capable of preserving what is best in community life: social co-responsibility, mutual aid, friendship among families. In this way, one can confidently state today that the plague which goes by the name of domestic violence, which afflicts thousands of children throughout Brazil every year, has been much reduced in families 'accompanied' by Pastoral Child-care. This is an effective way of preventing families from abandoning children, who then go out on to the streets in search of survival or an escape from a hostile family environment, swelling the ranks of 'street children'. There is no record of any child who has been 'accompanied' by Pastoral Child-care ending up on the streets.

Although it is difficult to measure the efficacy of the 'From Womb to Six' catechesis carried out by Pastoral Child-care, the joy and contentment of these children taking part in liturgical celebrations is plain to see, which shows that they are being influenced by cultural/religious values and by the experience of acting as a community.

The government itself has recognized the effective collaboration of Pastoral Child-care in eradicating poliomyelitis and measles, in the drastic reduction in cases of umbilical tetanus, whooping-cough, and diphtheria; not to mention the reduction in infant deaths from diarrhoea, perinatal fever and pneumonia, the three main causes of death in infants under one year old in Brazil; also its contribution to controlling other endemic regional diseases such as dengue, ulceration, malaria, and Hansen's disease. It is also concerned in preventing sexually-transmitted diseases such as AIDS, through counselling work with families and young people, working together with other pastoral and like agencies. Pastoral Child-care is always invited to take part in meetings and councils, which has also given it a voice in determining public policy.

Despite these successes, we need to bear in mind that solving the problems that condemn eleven per cent of the population of Brazil to live in absolute poverty requires an approach on two fronts. The first is a change on the macro-structural level of the country, so as to make possible a fairer distribution of income and better health and education for those who lack them. The second is an urgent coming-together of efforts by all sectors of society to reach those families in need, working with fathers, mothers, relatives and neighbours to find solutions capable of assuring an improvement in the quality of life of children, committing everyone in a new social ethic and in building a culture based on respect for and a proper evaluation of life.

The rescue of so many of our citizens and the need for all to have access to benefits that can no longer remain at the disposal of only a small section of society requires greater care of children from their mothers' wombs. They are the defenceless of today and the human resources of tomorrow and, as such, the greatest material and spiritual riches of families and the country.

Conclusion

Today, after fourteen years, I feel that every ounce of credibility gained by Pastoral Child-care, inside and outside the country, with scientific organizations, government and non-governmental agencies, has been won through the love and dedication, blood and sweat of thousands of women and men organized in small communities, learning, teaching, living the union of faith and life. I should like all communities to know this story, this experience of Christian love. I often ask myself: Why is it that so many parishes still do not implement our programmes? What is lacking to make all communities know and live this experience, if Jesus showed us the way and science confirms that the greatest changes can come only through changing human beings at the dawn of their lives? But we are also certain that this objective will one day be achieved. Pastoral Child-care is growing every year throughout the country.

It is also a great joy to learn that our experiences are beginning to be copied in several other countries in Latin America and in Africa. These experiences can be adapted to any country that seeks to combat poverty, domestic violence, maternal and infant mortality, by promoting life through working as a community, involving families through a leadership network that has been properly instructed and is committed to the cause.

The characteristics of seeking coordinators committed to Christian spirituality, effective sharing in the community, an ecumenical approach, well defined objectives, the system of empowering and accompanying, an information system to appraise results and identify problems, and the low cost of our activities, are all both necessary and responsible for the miracles that are worked every day in Pastoral Child-care – far more numerous than those recounted in the Bible, a real multiplying of loaves and fishes, which could be done in all communities in any country. Today I see clearly that the secret of these fourteen years of Pastoral Child-care has been to unfold, in the events of life, the experience of Christian love, which leads to the changes necessary for 'all to have life and have it in abundance' (John 10.10).

Translated by Paul Burns

Notes

1. According to research carried out by the World Health Organization, children oppressed in their first year of life have a marked tendency to violence and criminality. See OPS/WHO, *Mental Health and Psychosocial Development in Childhood: Basic Patterns and Proposals for an Inter-agency Action Plan at Regional Level*, nd.

2. The aim of Pastoral Child-care's sharing in social control is to empower leaders to take part in municipal bodies that control public services, such as town health councils, social services, education in the rights of children and adolescents. So as to make this participation possible, Pastoral Child-care has developed REBIDIA (*Rede Brasileira de Informaçao e Documentaçao sobre a Infância e Adolescência*, 'Brazilian network of information and documentation on childhood and adolescence'), with a Home Page on the Internet: http:/www.rebidia.org.br.

Contributors

JOHANN-BAPTIST METZ was born in 1928 in Auerbach (Bavaria), was ordained priest in 1954, holds doctorates in philosophy and theology, and is currently Professor of Fundamental Theology in the University of Münster. His publications include: *Asmut im Geist* (1962); *Christliche Anthropozentrik* (1962); *Zur Theologie der Welt* (1968) (ET *Theology of the World*, 1969); *Reform und Gegenreformation heute* (1969); *Kirche im Prozess der Aufklärung* (1970); *Die Theologie in der interdisziplinären Forschung* (1971); *Leidensgeschichte* (1973); *Unsere Hoffnung* (1975); *Zeit der Orden? Zur Mystik und Politik der Nachfolge* (1977); *Glaube in Geschichte und Gesellschaft* (1977) (ET *Faith in History and Society*, 1980); *Gott nach Auschwitz* (1979); *Jenseits bürgerlicher Religion* (1980); *Unterbrechungen* (1981); *Die Theologie der Befreiung – Hoffnung oder Gefahr für die Kirche?* (1986); *Zukunftsfähigkeit. Suchbewegungen im Christentum* (1987); *Lateinamerika und Europa: Dialog der Theologen* (1988); *Welches Christentum hat Zukunft?* (1990); *Gottespassion* (1991); *Augen für die Anderen* (1991).

Address: Kapitelstrasse 14, D 4400 Münster, Germany.

GASPAR MORA was born in Llavaneres in Catalonia in 1939. He studied at the seminary in Barcelona and at the Gregorian University and the Alphonsian Institute in Rome. He holds a doctorate in theology and teaches moral theology at the Theological Faculty of Catalonia in Barcelona. He is also an international counsellor in marriage preparation. His publications include *La carta a los Hebreos como escrito pastoral* (1974); *Praxis cristiana I* (collaborative, 1980); *L'estatut de la moral cristiana* (1983); *Fent camí amb les parelles* (1989); 'Etica sexual', in M. Vidal (ed.) *Conceptos fundamentales de ética teológica* (1992).

Address: Església 70, E-08950 Esplugues de Llobregat, Catalunya, Spain.

JOHN H. SIMPSON is Professor of Sociology and member, Centre for the Study of Religion, University of Toronto.

Address: 2351 Hargood Place, Mississauga, Ontario, Canada L5M 3G3.

JUNG MO SUNG was born in South Korea in 1957 and has lived in Brazil since 1966. A Catholic, married with two children, he holds degrees in philosophy and theology and doctorates in moral theology and science of religion. Specializing in the relationship between theology and economics, he lectures on post-graduate courses at the Catholic University of Sao Paulo and the Methodist Institute in S. Bernardo do Campo, besides overseeing Catholic communities and pastoral work and ecumenical movements. He has published six books, including *Idolatria do Capital e a morte dos pobres* (1989); *Deus numa economia sem coraçao: neoliberalismo e pobreza* (1992); *Teologia e economia: repensando a Teologia da Libertaçao e utopias* (1994).

Address: R. Humberto I, 254, Apto 121-A, 04018–030 Sao Paulo, Brazil.

HERMANN HÄRING was born in 1937 and studied theology in Munich and Tübingen; between 1969 and 1980 he worked at the Institute of Ecumenical Research in Tübingen; since 1980 he has been Professor of Dogmatic Theology at the Catholic University of Nijmegen. His books include *Kirche und Kerygma. Das Kirchenbild in der Bultmannschule* (1972); *Die Macht des Bösen. Das Erbe Augustins* (1979); *Zum Problem des Bosen in der Theologie* (1985); he was a co-editor of the *Wörterbuch des Christentums*, 1988, and has written articles on ecclesiology and christology, notably in the *Tijdschrift voor Theologie*.

Address: Katholieke Universiteit, Faculteit der Godgeleerdheid, Erasmusgebouw, Erasmusplein 1, 6525 HT Nijmegen, Netherlands.

PABLO RICHARD was born in Chile in 1939 and ordained a Catholic priest in 1967. He holds degrees in theology from the Catholic University of Chile (1966), in scriptural studies from the Pontifical Biblical Institute in Rome (1969), biblical archaeology from the Ecole Biblique in Jerusalem (1970), and has a doctorate in the sociology of religion from the Sorbonne in Paris (1978). He currently lectures in exegesis at the National University of Costa Rica and coordinates the education programme of the DEI (Ecumenical Research Department) in San José, dedicated to the permanent formation of pastoral agents in Latin America. The author of several books and numerous articles, his most recent publication is *Apocalypse: A People's Commentary on the Book of Revelation*.

Address: Departamento Ecumenico de Investigaciones, A.P. 389–2070 Sababilla, San José, Costa Rica.

ELSA TAMEZ was born in Mexico in 1950, of Mexican parents. She holds degrees in theology and in language and linguistics from Costa Rica and a doctorate in theology from the University of Lausanne. She has lectured in biblical theology at the Latin American Biblical Seminary in Costa Rica and been a member of the Ecumenical Research Department in San José. She is currently Rector of the Latin American Biblical Seminary. She is also a member of the Ecumenical Theological Education committee of the World Council of Churches, a moderator of EATWOT, and theological consultant to the Latin American Council of Churches. Her linguistic studies bore fruit in a *Concise Greek–Spanish Dictionary* (1987). Her works translated into English include *Bible of the Oppressed* (1979); *Through her Eyes: Women's Theology from Latin America* (1986); and *The Amnesty of Grace: Justification from a Latin American Perspective* (1991).

Address: Seminario Biblico Latinoamericano, Calle 3, Avenidas 14 y 16, Apdo. 901–1000, San José, Costa Rica.

JUSTIN S. UKPONG, a Catholic priest of the diocese of Uyo in Nigeria, is a professor of New Testament. He is Head of the Department of Biblical Studies at the Catholic Institute of West Africa, Port Harcourt, Nigeria, and the founding editor of the *Journal of Inculturation Theology*, the Institute's academic journal. He is currently the President of the Catholic Theological Association of Nigeria. His publications include *African Theologies Now – A Profile* (1984); *Sacrifice – African and Biblical: A Comparative Study of Ibibio and Levitical Sacrifices* (1987); *Gospel Parables in African Context* (ed., 1988); *Proclaiming the Kingdom: Essays in Contextual New Testament Studies* (1993); *Essays in Contextual Theology* (1995); and *New Testament Essays* (1995).

Address: Catholic Institute of West Africa, P.O. Box 499, Port Harcourt, Nigeria.

WALTER WINK is Professor of Biblical Interpretation at Auburn Theological Seminary in New York City. Previously he was a parish minister and taught at Union Theological Seminary in New York City. In 1989–1990 he was a Peace Fellow at the United States Institute for Peace. He is the author of a trilogy, *The Powers*, which consists of: *Naming the Powers: The Language of Power in the New Testament*, Philadelphia 1984; *Unmasking the Powers: The Invisible Forces that Determine Human Existence*, Philadelphia 1986; *Engaging the Powers: Discernment and Resistance in a World of Domination*, Minneapolis 1993. He has also written many other books, including *The Bible in Human Transformation*, Philadelphia 1973 and *Transforming Bible Study*, Nashville 1990.

Address: 155 Sandisfield Road, Sandisfield, MA 01755 USA.

NORBERT METTE was born in Barkhausen/porta, Germany, in 1946. After studying theology and sociology he gained a doctorate in theology, and since 1984 he has been Professor of Practical Theology at the University of Paderborn. He is married with three children. He has written numerous works on pastoral theology and religious education, including: *Voraussetzungen christlicher Elementarerziehung* (1983); *Kirche auf dern Weg ins Jahr 2000* (with M. Blasberg-Kuhnke, 1986); *Gemeindepraxis in Grundbegriffen* (with C. Bäumler, 1987); *Auf der Seite der Unterdrückten? Theologie der Befreiung im Kontext Europas* (ed. with P. Eicher, 1989); *Der Pastorale Notstand* (with O. Fuchs, 1992); *Religionspädagogik* (1994).

Address: Liebigweg 11a, D48165 Münster, Germany.

MARCIANO VIDAL was born in S. Pedro de Trones, in the León region of Spain. He is a priest of the Redemptorist Congregation and a doctor of theology specializing in moral theology. He lectures at the Pontifical University of Comillas in Madrid and is director of and lecturer at the Redemptorists' Higher Institute of Moral Sciences there. His major publication is the four-volume manual of theological ethics, *Moral de Actitudes*, now in its eighth edition (1995). His most recent publications are a study of the family in the life and thought of St Alphonsus de'Liguori (1995); an essay on conscientious objection (1995); an examination of the virtue and ethical principle of solidarity (1996); *La estimativa moral. Propuesto para la educación moral* (1997); and *Moral y espiritualidad* (1997). He is a director-counsellor member of the Board of Directors of *Concilium*.

Address: Manuel Silvela 14, 28010 Madrid, Spain.

ZILDA ARNS NEUMANN, founder and national coordinator of *Pastoral da Criança* (Pastoral Child-care), was born in 1934 in the Brazilian state of Santa Catarina. She obtained a degree in medicine from the Federal University of Paraná in 1959 and went on to specialize in: physical education (1961), pediatrics (1967), social pediatrics (1972), administration of mother-and-child health programmes (1975), public health for medical graduates (1977), and education in mother-and-child health (1977). In 1983 her brother, Cardinal Paulo Evaristo Arns of Sao Paulo, invited her to devise and head Pastoral Child-care, which functions as a 'social action organ' of the National Conference of Brazilian Bishops and represents it on the National Health Council. She has been invited to export her work at numerous events and has received a number of prizes and honourable mentions in Brazil and outside, such as the OPAS prize for Health Administration in 1994 and the conferral of the National Order of Merit for Education by the President of the Republic in October 1994.

Address: Pastoral da Criança, Rua Pasteur 279, Curutiba (PR), Brazil.

The editors wish to thank the great number of colleagues who contributed in a most helpful way to the final project.

K. Demmer	Rome	Italy
Z. M. Dias	Rio de Janeiro	Brazil
R. Gibellini	Brescia	Italy
T. Goffi†	Brescia	Italy
B. van Iersel	Nijmegen	The Netherlands
B. Kern	Mainz	Germany
H. Laubach	Mainz	Germany
M. Mette	Münster	Germany
J. Moltmann	Tübingen	Germany
G. Mora	Barcelona	Spain
M. O'Brien	Box Hill	Australia
T. Okure	Harcourt	Nigeria
H. Oppenheimer	Jersey	England
P. Richard	San José	Costa Rica
J. Riches	Glasgow	Scotland
A. Sanon	Bobo-Dioulasso	Burkina Faso
J. Ukpong	Harcourt	Nigeria

Members of the Board of Directors

Foundation

Anton van den Boogard	President	Nijmegen	The Netherlands
Paul Brand	Secretary	Ankeveen	The Netherlands
Werner Jeanrond		Lund	Sweden
Dietmar Mieth		Tübingen	Germany
Christoph Theobald SJ		Paris	France
Miklós Tomka		Budapest	Hungary

Founders

Anton van den Boogaard	Nijmegen	The Netherlands
Paul Brand	Ankeveen	The Netherlands
Yves Congar OP†	Paris	France
Hans Küng	Tübingen	Germany
Johann Baptist Metz	Vienna	Austria
Karl Rahner SJ†	Innsbruck	Austria
Edward Schillebeeckx OP	Nijmegen	The Netherlands

Directors-Counsellors

José Oscar Beozzo	São Paolo, SP	Brazil
Virgil Elizondo	San Antonio, TX	USA
Seán Freyne	Dublin	Ireland
Hermann Häring	Nijmegen	The Netherlands
Maureen Junker-Kenny	Dublin	Ireland
Werner Jeanrond	Lund	Sweden
François Kabasele Lumbala	Mbuji Mayi	Zaire
Karl-Josef Kuschel	Tübingen	Germany
Nicholas Lash	Cambridge	Great Britain
Dietmar Mieth	Tübingen	Germany
John Panagnopoulos	Athens	Greece
Giuseppe Ruggieri	Catania	Italy
Elisabeth Schüssler Fiorenza	Cambridge, MA	USA
Christoph Theobald SJ	Paris	France
Miklós Tomka	Budapest	Hungary
David Tracy	Chicago, IL	USA
Marciano Vidal CSSR	Madrid	Spain
Felix Wilfred	Madras	India
Ellen van Wolde	Tilburg	The Netherlands

General Secretariat: Prins Bernardstraat 2, 6521 A B Nijmegen, The Netherlands
Manager: Mrs E. C. Duindam-Deckers

CONCILIUM

The Theological Journal of the 1990s

Now available from Orbis Books

Founded in 1965 and published five times a year, *Concilium* is a world-wide journal of theology. Its editors and essayists encompass a veritable 'who's who' of theological scholars. Not only the greatest names in Catholic theology, but also exciting new voices from every part of the world, have written for this unique journal.

Concilium exists to promote theological discussion in the spirit of Vatican II, out of which it was born. It is a catholic journal in the widest sense: rooted firmly in the Catholic heritage, open to other Christian traditions and the world's faiths. Each issue of *Concilium* focusses on a theme of crucial importance and the widest possible concern for our time. With contributions from Asia, Africa, North and South America and Europe, *Concilium* truly reflects the multiple facets of the world church.

Now available from Orbis Books, *Concilium* will continue to focus theological debate and to challenge scholars and students alike.

Please enter my subscription to **Concilium** 1998/1-5

[ ] individual US$60.00   [ ] institutional US$75.00

Please send the following back issues at US$15.00 each

1996 . . . .   1995 . . . .

1994 . . . .   1993 . . . .

1992 . . . .   1991 . . . .

[ ] MC/Visa . . . . . . / . . . . . . / . . . . . . / . . . . . Expires . . . .

[ ] Check (payable to Orbis Books)

Name/Institution . . . .

Address . . . .

City/State/Zip . . . .

Telephone . . . .

Send order and payment to:
Orbis Books, Box 302, Maryknoll, NY 10545-0302 USA

Concilium Subscription Information - outside North America

Individual Annual Subscription (five issues): £25.00

Institution Annual Subscription (five issues): £35.00

Airmail subscriptions: add £10.00

Individual issues: £8.95 each

New subscribers please return this form:
for a two-year subscription, double the appropriate rate

(for individuals)   £25.00   (1/2 years)   . . . .

(for institutions)   £35.00   (1/2 years)   . . . .

Airmail postage
outside Europe +£10.00   (1/2 years)   . . . .

Total . . . .

I wish to subscribe for one/two years as an individual/institution
(delete as appropriate)

Name/Institution . . . .

Address . . . .

. . . .

. . . .

I enclose a cheque for . . . . payable to SCM Press Ltd

Please charge my Access/Visa/Mastercard no. . . . .

Signature . . . . Expiry Date . . . .

Please return this form to:
SCM PRESS LTD   9 - 17 St Albans Place   London   N1 0NX